MEDICAL
MINUTIAE

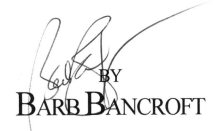

BY
BARB BANCROFT

□ WILLOWORKS PUBLISHING □

ISBN: 0-945115-02-4
Printed in the USA

Illustrations: Frank Salcido

A birth control method from our ancient Roman friends: Sneeze 3 times while leaping backward seven times after intercourse. The rationale of course, was that the abdominal muscle contractions caused by sneezing could push sperm out of the vagina.

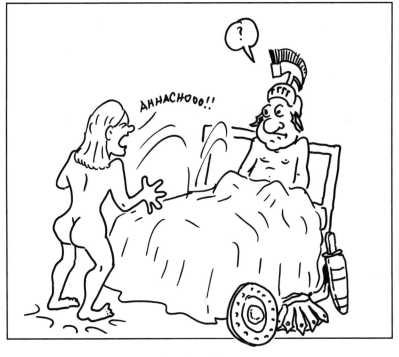

* * *

DISCLAIMER

This book is a collection of medical trivia. It is not intended to prescribe any kind of medical advice.

Neither the author, nor Willoworks Publishing shall be held liable, or responsible to any person for loss or damage caused, or said to be caused, directly or indirectly by ideas or information expressed in this book.

If you do not agree with this, or do not wish to be obliged to this agreement, please return this book (within 30 days of purchase) with the receipt to the publisher for a refund.

ACKNOWLEDGMENTS

To everyone with a sense of humor...

and thanks, Mom and Dad,
for giving me
such a great one.

TABLE OF

CONTENTS

NUTRITIONAL NUGGETS
1

A husband and wife eat grilled mahi-mahi, pasta, salad, water, and wine. Their pooch eats the leftovers. The husband and wife vomit. The pooch vomits. The husband and wife develop nausea, diarrhea, continued vomiting, headache, fever, rapid pulse—all within 45 minutes of their gourmet meal. The husband and wife and pooch improve with benadryl. What's the scoop?

This phenomenon is known as scromboid fish poisoning. Of all varieties of fish, the scromboid species (tuna, bonito, and mackerel) as well as dark meat fish, such as mahi-mahi, are most likely to develop high levels of histamine. When fresh scromboid fish is not continuously iced or refrigerated, bacteria may convert the amino acid histidine, which occurs naturally in the muscle of fish, to histamine. Since histamine is resistant to heat, cooking the fish generally will not prevent illness. In this instance the fish was imported from Taiwan through California, and shipped frozen to Albuquerque, NM where it was thawed and sold from a refrigerator case. Presumably, the lack of continuous freezing allowed the histadine conversion. The moral of the story—don't give your leftovers to your dog.

* * *

Do you have a meat fetish, but feel guilty about it? Here are six "skinniest" cuts of meat: eye of round, round tip, top loin, top round, sirloin, and tenderloin.

* * *

Ginger root has been used for thousands of years in Chinese herbal medicine to remedy nausea, vomiting, diarrhea, and abdominal pain—just to name a few ailments. In actual tests, ginger root was found to be superior to Dramamine, an anti-cholinergic drug used in the prevention and treatment of motion sickness. Ginger has also been shown to have anti-coagulant properties.

* * *

After gulping down your morning dose of ginger root, toss down ten cloves of garlic. Garlic has been used for over 5,000 years as a cure for any number of ailments. Ancient Romans used it for 61 different maladies. It has antibiotic, anti-viral, immune stimulation, anti-hypertensive, anti-coagulant, and anti-carcinogenic properties. Just looking at the list would make you tend to believe that garlic is the cure-all for anything that ails ya'. However, the thought of belting down ten or more cloves of garlic a day to prevent cancer, makes the thought of apples, oat bran, and fiber much more appetizing.

Garlic has been shown to lower LDLs, VLDLs cholesterol, and triglyceride levels as well as raise the protective levels of HDLs (good cholesterol). However, this positive effect was observed only after an individual had consumed 10 cloves of garlic per day for 6 months. One may wonder how anyone got close enough to draw serum levels on this particular group of patients completing the study.

Not only has garlic been shown to have a protective effect on the development of arteriosclerosis (possibly), it has also been shown to release substances that have an anti-tumor effect.

The active garlic ingredient is diallyl sulfide. Mice were fed this extract of garlic prior to exposure to a known colorectal carcinogen. Results of the study showed 75% less tumors in the group with the garlic compound vs. the control group without the garlic compound. Similar studies were performed with esophageal cancers and found a 100% difference.

* * *

How about an onion for coronary artery disease? One half of a raw onion will boost HDL levels in about two-thirds of the patients who have the guts to chomp on a raw onion, and who have the ability to cope with the lack of close friends and relationships. The onion must be raw, not cooked, to have the beneficial effect.

* * *

Speaking of cholesterol...soon after exercising, the blood level of cholesterol actually rises by about 10-15%. Thus, if one works out, runs, or goes for a long walk in the morning prior to giving blood for cholesterol determination, the level will be misleadingly high.

*　　*　　*

Ever wondered why that steaming bowl of chicken noodle soup always helped when you had a stuffy, itchy nose, fever, and "generalized malaise"? Well, the therapeutic benefits from a bowl of steaming, piping hot chicken noodle soup have

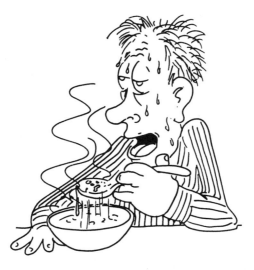

finally been tested in a controlled trial, and it all boils down to the steam and NOT the chicken noodle soup. Two groups of thirty-one patients with common colds were asked to refrain from taking cold medications. One group was treated with a specially designed device that produced a constant flow of water-saturated hot (105°F) air (a fancy term for steam), and the other group used a placebo machine—one that blew unmoisturized room-temperature air. Each patient received two 20-minute treatments during a period of approximately two hours.

Symptoms of both groups improved over a seven day period—as you would expect with any common cold. However, the steam-treated group had a far greater improvement in symptoms—81% of the group using steam had improvements vs. only 23% who used the drier room air. Also, measurements of air flow through the nose on the morning after treatment improved in approximately 70% of those who used steam.

The basis for the benefit of steam remains to be clarified, however, it may be related to the fact that viral proliferation is impaired as temperature increases.

*   *   *

To keep the dentist away, eat a chunk of cheese after you finish a meal. At least twelve different types of cheese,

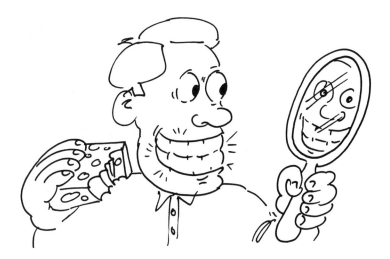

including cheddar, mozzarella, Edam, and Gouda neutralize acids in saliva and help to prevent tooth decay. Aged cheddar has also been shown to replenish enamel in decay-weakened tooth surfaces.

*   *   *

Americans go through 700 million pounds of peanut butter each year. This gummy spread was first discovered in the early 1900s by a St. Louis physician who wanted to make a high protein diet supplement for his elderly patients who were unable to chew meat. In fact, a sandwich-size 3-tablespoon serving of peanut butter contains 13.5 grams of protein—about the amount in 2 eggs or a 12-oz. glass of milk. Three tablespoons also contains 4 grams of fiber—about as much as in a couple of slices of whole wheat bread. The downside: 3 tablespoons of peanut butter equals 300 calories.

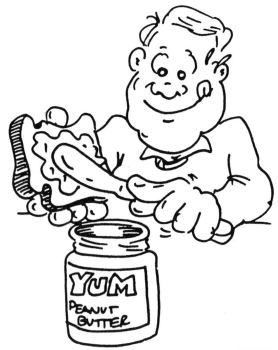

Q. Why does peanut butter stick to the roof of your mouth?

A. The high concentration of protein gives it an incredible ability to absorb and hold moisture—in other words, it sops up your saliva.

* * *

In the early 60s and 70s, the fiber rich bran from wheat was fed to cattle. What happened? We were constipated and the cows were regular.

* * *

The average American eats 1,148 pounds of food per year, including 117 pounds of potatoes, 128 pounds of beef, 100 pounds of veggies, 80 pounds of fresh fruits, and 286 eggs.

If you want to cut down on the number of eggs you eat per year, switch to ostrich eggs. The switch may not help your cholesterol level; however one ostrich egg will make 11½ omelets, so you definitely will cut down on the number of total eggs consumed.

* * *

Until late 1987 the Quaker Oats company was selling approximately one million boxes of oat bran cereal per year. Enter the oat bran craze to reduce cholesterol. Quaker Oats company now sells *one million boxes* of oat bran cereal *per month.*

* * *

What are the four predominant flavors in Juicy Fruit gum? Lemon, orange, pineapple, and banana...betcha didn't know that one.

* * *

Why is it that when you tell patients that two tablespoons of oat bran is good for you they will automatically assume that five or six tablespoons would obviously be much better for you? Well, one 75-year-old man did just that—he started taking 60 grams (about six heaped tablespoons full or one cupful) of oat bran daily in the form of bran muffins. He did this for approximately one week when he noticed that he hadn't had a bowel movement for several days. He arrived at the emergency room with abdominal pain and bloating. He was transferred to the operating room with the diagnosis of an intestinal obstruction. Surgery was performed for the intestinal obstruction with cancer listed as the probable cause. Instead of a large cancerous tumor blocking his sigmoid colon, the surgeon found a 2-foot-long column of oat bran. Too much oat bran had overwhelmed the ability of the intestinal muscles to move it along—hence, the obstruction.

*　*　*

And speaking of obstructions, here's another one for you. Abdominal surgery was performed on a woman with the clinical diagnosis of intestinal obstruction. Since the woman was older it was presumed to be a mass produced by a tumor. However, a tumor was not the cause of the blockage. Instead, she had a complete undigested apricot blocking the lumen of the intestine. How, you might ask, could this happen, especially since it would be tough to swallow an apricot in its entirety? The woman's daughter mentioned that she had given her Mom some dried fruit several days before. Could it be that the dried fruit absorbed the water and expanded into a mass blocking the bowel? As an experiment, the patient's doctor soaked some dried apricots in water for twenty-four hours and found that this produced what appeared to be some fresh whole apricots about the size of golf balls. She probably did not chew her dried food properly and swallowed it whole. So the moral of the story is: "Chew your food, dear, especially if it is dried fruit."

* * *

Most hard-boiled eggs end up with off-center yolks. This is why deviled eggs have defied automation for all these years.

* * *

Researchers at New Mexico University suggest that we start eating tumbleweed. Right. They claim that it is fairly nutritious and can be turned into vitamins and food additives. A bonus use for tumbleweed fibers—they can be used for the production of sanitary napkins. For some reason that thought doesn't seem to be a comfortable one. Would you call them Prairie Pads?

* * *

Did you know that the quality and flavor of cheese is inversely proportional to the thickness of the slice? So when that tightwad neighbor of yours served you those wafer-thin slices of cheese and you rudely thought to yourself, "What a cheapskate," he (she) was actually enhancing your taste buds, unbeknownst to you, the uninformed Philistine.

* * *

The weight loss clinic at Duke University prescribes pump sprays of your favorite cravings—in other words, when the overwhelming urge for an apple-cinnamon Danish hits, you can whip out your handy-dandy pump spray and give yourself a squirt for only one-tenth of a calorie per squirt. This seems to satisfy that overpowering desire for the apple-cinnamon

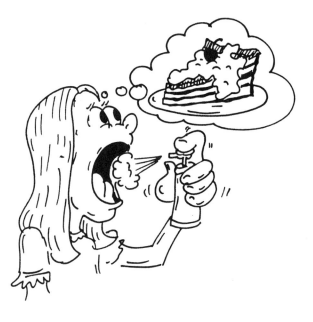

Danish, but what about the pizza attack that arrives two hours later? Yes, a pump spray has also been produced with the pepperoni-mozzarella cheese aroma. Others include chocolate, peanut butter, grape jelly, butterscotch, and potato chip flavors.

*   *   *

One ton of grapes will make 170 gallons of wine.

*   *   *

American women spent almost 260 million bucks on girdles in 1992, almost 10 million more than in 1982. By the way, the term girdle is considered archaic these days. Sounds rather old-fashioned and nerdy to wear a girdle so we now wear "molders," "shapers," "smoothers," or "trimmers." Although the name has changed to protect the innocent, the function still remains the same—to hide our bulges, blubber, and excess flab.

*   *   *

Almost 48 million Americans dine on fast- food per day: 5.2 billion hamburgers and cheeseburgers are consumed per year, or 198.4 million in a typical two week period. Gross sales for fast-food in 1986 totaled 51.2 million dollars. There are more than 120,000 fast-food restaurants in the United States. Singles, men, and two-income families are most likely to chow down at fast-food restaurants.

For those of you who consider yourself a fast-food fanatic, such as myself, take a look at some of the things you eat, and what they contain. These are some of my favorites:

Wendy's Double Burger: Calories 560, Sodium 575 mg. (Compare this to a Big Mac attack: 563 calories and sodium 1,010 mg.)

McDonald's McNuggets (6): Calories 314, Sodium 525 mg. (Compare this to KFC nuggets with 262 calories and 810 mg sodium.)

McDonald's Fries: Calories 220, Sodium 109 mg. (Compare to Wendy's fries with 280 calories and 95 mg sodium.)

Choose your excess poundage wisely and tastefully. Know your fast-foods. And also know where you can buy the inevitable "trimmer," "molder," "shaper," or "smoother," or just borrow Mom's girdle.

*   *   *

Each person in the U.S. consumes, on the average, 128 pounds of potatoes each year. Five billion pounds of U.S. potatoes become French fries each year, thanks to our ever-growing hunger for fast-food restaurants. The first potato arrived on U.S. soil in 1622 as a gift from Bermuda. We can thank Thomas Jefferson for the first French fry—he brought them home from Paris in the late 1700s.

Another use for a potato—to escape from jail. John Dillinger reportedly carved a gun from a potato and turned it black with iodine.

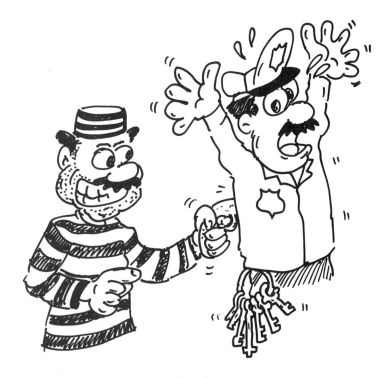

*   *   *

How many of you are Spam (combination "spiced" and "ham") lovers? Well, if you are, this info is for you. Spam consists of a loaf of molded ground pork shoulder with some added ground ham, salt, H_2O, sugar, and sodium nitrite. The amount of sodium in one 2-oz. serving of Spam is enough to make even the strongest heart quiver: it contains 1,724 mg of sodium, 170 calories, and 30 grams of fat. So Spam's not high on the list of dietetic foods either.

Spam is manufactured by the George A. Hormel Company of Austin, Minnesota and at this very moment it controls 75% of the canned luncheon meat market. That's amazing to me. How many of your closest friends chow down on a Spam and cheese sandwich? Someone must do it on the sly, because 85 million pounds of canned Spam are sold per year.

And, how about those Pork Packers of the world? Did you know they had a Journal called *Squeal?* (Is that not a wonderful name? Not only is the name great, but doesn't it amaze you that the Pork Packers of the world have a journal???) Anyway, an article in *Squeal* called the introduction of Spam as "historic" as the first rifle shot at the Battle of Lexington. No doubt they are the only ones to make this analogy. In the "What's on the Menu" section of the journal, the following recipes were found: Polynesian Baked Spam, Sweet and Sour Spam, Spam enchilada breakfast Casserole, and Spaghetti Carbonara with Spam, not to mention the cool Spam, cucumber, and avocado sandwiches for the politically correct.

* * *

Nutritionists at the University of Columbia in Missouri have found that buying extra lean ground beef for the purposes of reducing dietary fat and cholesterol is a waste of money. In comparing broiled burgers made from 100 grams of regular, lean, and extra lean ground beef, they found that the cholesterol levels were similar in all three types after cooking. In addition, the fat content of all three types varied only 5% after cooking, whereas in the pre-cooked state the variance was as great as 20%.

* * *

Constipated? Bad gums? Lousy teeth? Eat one to two quarts of popcorn per day for a safe, inexpensive remedy for all that ails ya'.

Americans are the largest per capita consumers of popcorn in the world. Over 10 BILLION quarts of popcorn are consumed per year, grossing over 1 billion dollars for the popcorn industry.

* * *

Each year Americans drink about 127 billion cups of coffee. Twenty-five percent of those cups are decaffeinated. Speaking of caffeine:
- drip coffee contains 150 mg per 5-ounce cup
- percolated coffee contains 100 mg per 5-ounce cup
- decaffeinated coffee contains 3 mg per 5-ounce cup

* * *

The most disliked foods in America:
1) tofu
2) liver
3) yogurt
4) Brussels sprouts
5) lamb
6) prunes

* * *

This question has boggled the masses for decades: Why are some pistachios dyed red? Pistachios were first mass-marketed in the U.S. in the 1930s during the Great Depression. At that time they were placed in vending machines mixed with the bland cashew and the pallid peanut. Some ingenious pistachio manufacturer decided that he would dye them red to make them stand out in the crowd. It worked and pistachios became a hit.

* * *

The average American consumes 1,417 pounds of food each year. Of that, nine pounds are chemical additives.

* * *

The average American (do you ever wonder who the average American is?) ate 9.7 pounds of pasta in 1975 versus 15.4 pounds in 1992.

* * *

Free radicals are a group of chemicals produced by various bodily biochemical processes. Most researchers agree that these free radicals (also known as oxidants) are responsible for the cellular destruction involved in various inflammatory systemic diseases such as rheumatoid arthritis, as well as in the aging process such as cataract formation. It would make perfectly good sense to fight these free radicals with antioxidants, and nutritional research is heading in that direction.

Interestingly enough, many of us consume antioxidants in our daily diets. Vitamins C and E, selenium (concentrated in seafood, sunflower seeds, and nuts), and beta carotene (yellow-orange fruits and vegetables, and green leafy vegetables) are all antioxidants.

One of the most convincing arguments for the powers of antioxidants comes from a new study of Canadians over the age of 55. It found that those who had taken Vitamin C (at least 300 mg daily) for the previous 5 years had 70% lower risk of cataracts than non-vitamin C users. A daily vitamin E capsule (400 IU) also cut the cataract risk in half.

By the way, cigarette smoking increases free radical formation in the lens of the eye. For this reason, cigarette smoking is associated with a much higher risk of cataract formation.

Fish oil also contains antioxidants. Diets high in fish oil have been shown to be beneficial for some patients with rheumatoid arthritis.

* * *

Is your microwave or oven on the blink? One Massachusetts couple found that their salmon was too large to

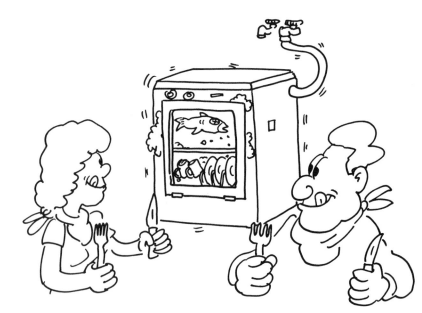

fit in a steamer so they wrapped it in a cheesecloth, placed it on a dish towel, and cooked it on the top rack of the dishwasher for one cycle. Potatoes take about the same time as salmon (one cycle and sometimes a second rinse). Peas do nicely with just a few minutes of the second rinse.

*   *   *

It may come as a shock to you, but there is no such fish as a sardine. The term "sardine" is actually a generic name for quite a number of different small fish. A small fish doesn't become a sardine until it has been canned. During the canning process certain oils, brines, and sauces are added which give the small fish their characteristic sardine flavor. Without these additives, sardines would not be palatable to most of us.

*   *   *

Peanut M&M's ranked #1 among all candies sold at New York City subway stands. Speaking of M&M's...an extremely important study was released in 1984 that revealed some fascinating findings about them:

- The average number of M&M's per standard package is 57, give or take one or two.
- Of that number, 33% were dark brown
- 25% were yellow
- 19% were orange
- 14% were light brown
- 9% were green.

Since green M&M's have the distinct reputation of being a powerful aphrodisiac, one wonders if the Mars-M&M company has lost its libido. One last pearl gleaned from the study is that each one of those tiny little morsels has an average of 4.2 calories.

*   *   *

The bad news...the average person is likely to ingest several grams of mutagens and carcinogens in food each day. Such common foods as alfalfa sprouts, tomatoes, potatoes, rhubarb, chocolate (I can't believe it!), herbal teas, celery, and mushrooms all contain material known to cause gene damage.

The good news...certain dietary foods, including whole grain cereals, citrus fruits, dark green veggies, deep yellow vegetables, and members of the family Cruciferae (broccoli, cabbage, cauliflower, and Brussels sprouts), all contain substances that inhibit the formation of cancer-causing chemicals or reduce cancer incidence in other ways.

*   *   *

Osteoporosis Update: Contrary to what one would expect, osteoporosis is most prevalent in affluent countries in which the consumption of dairy products, and consequently calcium, is high. Why the paradox? One reason may be the high protein intake that also occurs in affluent countries. Numerous studies have demonstrated that high protein intake promotes excessive calcium loss because excess protein is converted to urea and eliminated along with other mineral products. Animal protein has been shown to be more effective than vegetable protein in promoting calcium loss. In addition, affluent countries have a high intake of carbonated beverages which contain large amounts of phosphates believed to promote calcium loss. Increased amounts of sodium contained in processed foods also promote calcium loss. Excess sodium in the diet requires the elimination of large amounts of sodium in the urine, which also promotes the loss of other minerals such as calcium.

*   *   *

The number of quarts of ice cream consumed by the average Southerner each year is 12. The average New Englander consumes an average of 23 quarts per year.

*   *   *

Four days after quitting smoking, a person retains 46% more caffeine from a cup of coffee. Why? Cigarette smoking speeds the breakdown of caffeine in the blood, so that smokers need to drink more coffee to maintain their caffeine high.

*   *   *

Two sticks of licorice per day for seven days may result in a weight gain of one to five pounds. Licorice contains an aldosterone-like substance that causes sodium and water retention. This retention can lead to hypertension with headaches, vomiting, and photophobia. This has also been referred to as "Halloween Hypertension" —primarily seen in children during the week or two after Halloween.

*   *   *

Speaking of salt, one ounce of Cheerios for breakfast provides 333 mg of salt in your daily diet. Some of you may be breathing a sigh of relief, saying ,"Whew, I don't eat those salt-laden Cheerios, I eat Wheaties, the Breakfast of Champions!" Sorry to burst your cereal bowl, Wheaties have even more. One ounce of Wheaties provides 370 mg of salt.

And, by the way, have you noticed how much sodium one of those Lean Cuisine's contains?

*   *   *

That old wive's tale about drinking a glass of milk prior to bedtime actually has a biologic basis in helping the insomniacs of the world fall asleep. Yet, contrary to popular belief, you should not heat the milk! Milk appears to contain a natural hypnotic, L-tryptophan, the precursor to serotonin which is a neurotransmitter believed to help one sleep. Heating the milk may inactivate the L-tryptophan, therefore the natural effect would be negated.

* * *

Did you know that our federal government has passed legislation that regulates the flow of ketchup? It has been mandated that more than 9 cm. per 30 seconds is against the law. Finally, all those anxiety ridden, ketchup-flow legislators can now direct their energies to bigger and better things, which sure makes me anxious.

* * *

Americans drink the equivalent of 416 cans of soda for every man, woman, and child in the United States. It has been estimated that if every drop of Coke ever manufactured were to replace the water flowing over Niagara Falls, the soda would last for 16 hours and 48 minutes.

* * *

The use of food as medicine, especially preventative medicine, is making a dramatic comeback after nearly 5,000 years of use followed by a recent century of neglect. However, food does not replace modern drugs, as some would have you believe. The effects of food are more subtle, more slow-acting, and certainly more variable and difficult to gauge. What are some of these foods and what do they contain?

Patients with chronic bronchitis, sinus problems, colds, asthma, and emphysema may benefit from hot spicy foods such as jalapeños, hot sauce, horseradish, and garlic. These hot spices, such as capsaicin found in hot peppers, contain "mucokinetic" properties. They help to break up mucous and propel it up and out of the bronchi—much the same as Robitussin DM.

Oat bran and cholestyramine appear to have similar mechanisms of action. They both act as bile acid binding resins which attach to cholesterol in the intestine and move it down the line. Cholesterol is unable to be reabsorbed back into the serum and the levels will fall by as much as 20% in 85% of individuals. Legumes work in a similar way.

Citrus fruits are believed to have anti-cancer effects as well. National Cancer Institute studies have shown that people eating high amounts of citrus fruits, such as grapefruits, have lower rates of certain cancers. It is believed that Vitamin C is the major cancer antagonist.

Yogurt contains seven antibiotics, which aid in the control of GI infections and help to replenish the GI flora.

The *Edinburgh Journal* of 1859 promoted strong coffee as the treatment for asthma. The caffeine in coffee is a potent bronchodilator. Italian researchers found that the caffeine in three cups of coffee had the same bronchodilating effect as a standard dose of theophylline. They also found asthma to be less prevalent among coffee drinkers than non-coffee drinkers.

If you think all of this is a bunch of baloney, think back to your high-school history courses and the thousands of British sailors who died of the dreaded disease scurvy. It wasn't until the 18th century that a Scottish naval surgeon recommended a teaspoon or two of lime or lemon juice to prevent the disease. No one believed the doctor and it took more than 40 years to convince the British Navy to carry daily rations of citrus fruit. In the meantime, 200,000 sailors died of this totally preventable disease.

Omega-3 acids from fish oil have been shown to modify prostaglandins. Modifying prostaglandins helps to reduce the inflammatory response. Some researchers have shown that inflammation helps contribute to the formation of atherosclerotic plaques in the arteries. Therefore, two or three helpings of fish per week is advised.

Cruciferous vegetables (broccoli, cauliflower, Brussel sprouts, cabbage) appear to have an anti-carcinogenic effect in the lower intestinal tract. This was known by the folks that lived in ancient Rome—one group of ancient villagers banished all physicians, saying that they preferred to eat cabbages to stay healthy.

Fruits may have an effect on reducing the incidence of pancreatic cancer. A recent National Cancer Institute study in Southern Louisiana, where the rate of pancreatic cancer is high, suggests that eating fruit might help negate the carcinogenic effect of nitrates, such as bacon and other forms of pork.

A 1987 study from the Johns Hopkins School of Hygiene and Public Health found that people with the lowest levels of beta carotene were four times more likely to develop squamous cell carcinoma of the lung. One cooked carrot a day might cut the risk of developing lung cancer, especially among former smokers. Beta carotene acts as an antioxidant, which means it helps to protect cells from highly reactive chemicals called free radicals. Free radicals have been linked to cancer, heart disease, cataracts, aging, and rheumatoid arthritis.

A chemical factor in cranberry juice blocks the adherance of urinary tract pathogens to the bladder wall. Hence, the old wive's tale that cranberry juice prevents lower urinary tract infections.

*　　*　　*

The typical diet in China contains one-half the fat of the recommended U.S. diet. In other words, approximately 15% of the total calories in the Chinese diet are from fat sources. Fiber is three times more plentiful, and cholesterol levels are so low

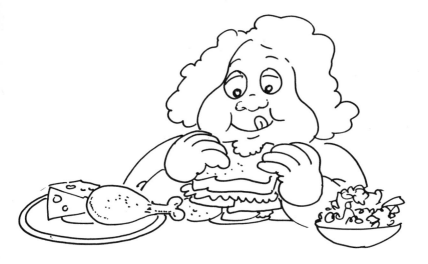

that they barely register on the serum cholesterol scales designed for the U.S. population. In addition, the Chinese consume approximately 20% more calories than we do, but there is very little obesity.

The incidence of coronary artery disease and colon cancer is negligible in the Chinese population. On the other hand, the incidence of hemorrhagic stroke is six times higher due to the low cholesterol levels. Remember that cholesterol is essential for the maintenance of the integrity of the blood vessel walls.

*   *   *

Spicy food stimulates perspiration. The perspiration produced by eating these foods evaporates on the skin producing a temporary cooling effect. This explains why people

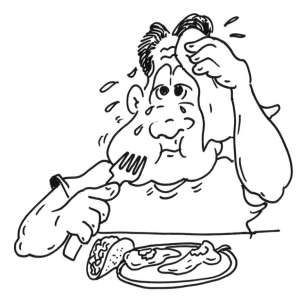

who live in hot places such as Mexico and India favor spicy foods such as hot peppers and curries.

*   *   *

Another reason to breast feed—it saves on orthodontist bills. Researchers at Johns Hopkins University School of Public

Health found that breast-fed babies use their mouth muscles more effectively when getting milk and are less likely than bottle-fed babies to end up with crooked teeth.

* * *

Listeria monocytogenes may be lurking in your refrigerator. Two new studies implicate bacteria-contaminated food can cause listeriosis, a rare, but potentially lethal illness in pregnant women, the elderly, and immunoincompetent patients. One of the studies found 64% of the refrigerators of patients with listeriosis had at least one edible item contaminated with *listeria monocytogenes*. Foods such as lunch meat, cheese (especially soft cheeses such as feta) and leftovers, contained the bacteria. Most people with healthy immune systems don't have to worry about listeriosis, however those mentioned above should avoid deli meats, soft cheeses, and should reheat leftovers until they are steaming hot. (*JAMA*, April 15, 1992)

* * *

During WWII, pilots were fed huge amounts of carotene to improve their night vision. Many pilots developed carotenemia, an orange-like discoloration of the skin, and indication of beta carotene excess. Some individuals might mistake this skin discoloration for jaundice; however, with carotenemia the sclera (the white membrane covering the eyeball) are not discolored.

* * *

Dentists have found yet another reason for us to remove the high fat intake from our diets. People who indulge in greasy and creamy foods get more cavities. The reason seems to be an elevated level of fatty substances in their saliva. Switching to a low-fat diet solves the problem.

* * *

You have always heard that eating small amounts six times a day is much better for you than eating all of your calories in three meals per day, but you never heard why. The snack advantage may be due to food's effect on insulin secretin from the pancreas. The body releases insulin to counteract the rise in blood sugar following a meal. Large meals result in a dramatic boost of insulin that is large enough to stimulate the liver to produce cholesterol. It appears that by eating smaller meals cholesterol may be lowered.

* * *

The Human Nutrition Center in Beltsville, Maryland, recently reported that daily cinnamon in the diet can reduce the amount of insulin required for glucose breakdown. In addition, it can be cooked without breakdown of its main active ingredient, cinnamaldehyde.

* * *

Don't eat moldy cheese—it could be toxic. Those colored olive green or forest green appear to be the most toxic. Least toxic are shades of blue, gray and bluish green. Certain cheeses however, are ripened with harmless molds that create bluish green veins or whitish felt rinds, such as bleu cheese, Stilton, Brie, and Camembert. Those cheeses are harmless. One misconception: Since the above cheeses are ripened with mold some people think that perhaps the resulting mold contains penicillin. Wrong. Most cheese molds can't make

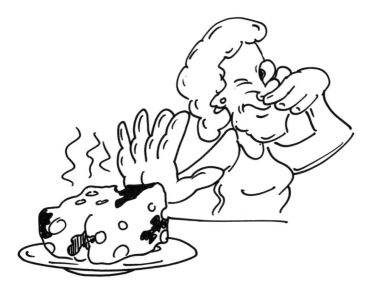

penicillin, so eat all the blue cheese you want, even if you're allergic to penicillin.

*   *   *

Celery may have beneficial health effects. A substance in celery, 3-n-butylphthalide, reduces the production of catecholamines and subsequently blood pressure. When University of Chicago investigators fed laboratory rats the equivalent of two large stalks of celery per day, their systolic blood pressure dropped an average of 12 to 14 percent and their cholesterol levels decreased about seven points. This remedy for hypertension has been touted in Asian medical lore for centuries—they recommended two stalks of celery per day. (P.S. Celery also contains sodium, so salt-sensitive individuals should use caution before they start munching on celery to reduce blood pressure.)

*   *   *

Microwaving breast milk reduces the protective effect of IgA maternal antibodies by 79%. In addition, the activity of lysozymes (enzymes that destroy pathogens) is reduced by 19%. Any temperature above 140° F can produce these effects. Moral of the story: heat it the old fashioned way.

* * *

EAT YOGURT—IT'S GOOD FOR YA'

1) Yogurt is high in calcium, it also increases the acidic gastrointestinal pH thereby increasing calcium absorption.

2) Yogurt contains protective bacteria that colonize the GI tract and vagina; this colonization weakens pathogenic bacteria.

3) A February 25, 1992 study in the *Annals of Internal Medicine* found that yogurt reduced the incidence of vaginitis in women who had recurrent yeast infection. The yogurt used contained two types of bacteria—*lactobacillus bulgaricus* and *streptococcus thermophilus*. Another beneficial bacteria is *lactobacillus acidophilus*, added to some milk products, and also available in tablets, capsules, and powder form to assist in lactose digestion. Yogurt that is pasteurized loses its beneficial effects. The process of pasteurization kills all three of the above bacteria in milk or yogurt products. Look for labels that state "live cultures" or "non-pasteurized." Frozen yogurt may also contain the bacteria, depending on the length of its storage in the freezer. The longer it is frozen, the more bacteria are killed.

Back to the study. Half of the women in the study ate one cup of yogurt daily for six months containing live cultures of *lactobacillus acidophilus*. The others consumed no yogurt for the same time period. After six months of this regimen, the groups switched for the next six months. During the yogurt-free phase of the trial, participants averaged three yeast infections each, however during the yogurt-phase, the rate of infection dropped to less than one per person.

*   *   *

What are the five most common foods causing asphyxiation in children?
- hot dogs
- candy
- peanuts
- grapes
- cookies/biscuits/other meats

*   *   *

Since yams contain estrogen, can post-menopausal females consume a healthy portion of yams per day in lieu of Premarin? Well, the answer is yes and no. First of all, one must eat abundant quantities of UNCOOKED yams. Cooking inactivates the estrogenic biologic activity in yams. In addition, even though there is an extremely small amount of estrogenic activity in one yam, estrogenic activity varies from yam to yam, and estrogenic activity varies from crop to crop. Therefore, it is very difficult to recommend a specific number of yams for daily estrogen replacement. Inadequate doses will not alleviate hot flashes, vaginal dryness, or osteoporosis, and excessive doses will cause nausea, anorexia, diarrhea, and thrombotic complications. Unopposed estrogens (those not opposed by the other female hormone, Progesterone) can cause uterine cancer.

Historically, yams were used to manufacture estrogen for human as well as animal use. Today we use urine from pregnant mares as a cheaper and more abundant source, hence the name of the drug—Premarin (**pregnant mares urine**). Plants also contain chemicals with estrogen-like activity. A report in the 1954 *Journal of Biochemistry* discussed the effects of large amounts of uncooked subterranean clover used to feed Australian sheep. The clover contained estrogen-like chemicals and caused sterility due to the large amounts ingested.

*   *   *

Gustatory rhinitis, otherwise known as the "salsa sniffles," occurs when one snarfs down meals containing chili

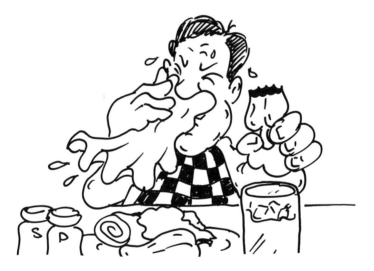

peppers, horseradish, onions, and other spicy hot food. These sniffles and drips are due to overstimulated parasympathetic (cholinergic) nerves that supply the glands located in the nasal passages. Fluid production is turned on and the drip begins. Researchers at the National Institute of Allergy and Infectious Diseases have developed a nasal spray containing an anti-cholinergic drug known as atropine. Just a squirt in each nostril prior to the hot spicy meals keeps noses dry 100% of the time. Side effects are nil.

* * *

Some patients have acne flare-ups when they eat various types of nuts. Keep in mind that this includes any foods cooked in peanut oil.

* * *

Pound for pound, chicken is 200 times more likely to cause illness than seafood (except shellfish) and 100 times more likely to result in death. However, raw and under-cooked shellfish are 100 times more likely to cause illness than chicken and 250 times more likely to result in death.

* * *

A recent issue of *Lancet* (1991; 338:899) reports on a Norwegian study's findings on the benefits of a vegetarian gluten-free diet and the abatement of symptoms in rheumatoid arthritis patients.

* * *

Is sushi safe to eat? Yes, but only if you eat it at a reputable Japanese restaurant. The problem happens to be parasitic tapeworms and roundworms that infect mackerel, tuna, and salmon. If the infected fish is eaten, the larvae may attach to the gastrointestinal tract lining and cause pain, nausea, and vomiting. Smoked salmon used in sushi bars is cold smoked—this process does not kill parasites.

Well-trained sushi chefs can eyeball the white BB-size cysts of tapeworms, and the thin spaghetti-like shape of roundworms. Your best friend trying to make sushi at home may not be able to spot the worms; therefore, homemade sushi is more likely to cause problems.

One type of tapeworm, known as *Diphyllobothrium* to its friends, is a particular nuisance to the human GI tract. Carried in larval cysts by Alaskan salmon, the worm attaches itself to the ileum and can grow ten to fifteen feet in length. This worm also competes with the human host for a variety of nutrients, B12 being the most important. An unexplained B12 deficiency anemia in a sushi fanatic may be caused by this culprit. The patient would also have GI complaints such as nausea, pain, and alternating diarrhea and constipation.

* * *

Can tea cause anemia? Yes. Tea drinking reduces the absorption of iron from the GI tract. A study performed in Israel evaluated 122 infants, aged 6-12 months. The percentage of tea-drinking infants with iron-deficiency anemia was 32.6% compared to 3.5% for the non-tea drinkers in the group. The tea drinkers had significantly lower hemoglobins as well. (Am J Clin Nutri 1985; 41: 1210)

* * *

Speaking of iron-deficiency anemia, it is the most common cause of a specific physical finding—blue sclera (the white part of the eye)—in adults and in children. Other causes of blue sclera include osteogenesis imperfecta, corticosteroid use, collagen disorders, and myasthenia gravis.

* * *

A University of Oregon study followed multiple sclerosis patients on an unsaturated fat diet for 34 years. Ninety-five percent of those who stayed with the unsaturated fat/no saturated fat diet were still alive and remained physically active at the end of the three decade period, even though the expected rate of MS patients doing well 34 years after diagnosis is only 4%. Of those who did not stay on the diet, 83% died and most survivors became disabled. The diet was similar to that used for cholesterol control—fish, chicken (white meat only), and vegetable fats were used instead of animal fats.

* * *

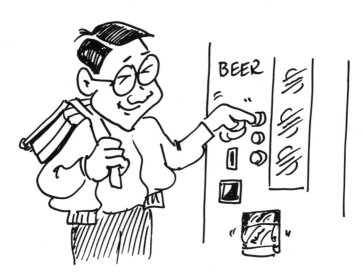

Beer is available from vending machines in Japan. Even though the legal drinking age is 20, one in every eight Japanese high school students, ages 16-18, were found to have a drinking problem in 1991. Just ten years ago the rate was one per one hundred.

* * *

The *New England Journal of Medicine* (323; 160:1990) published a report by South African researchers on the benefits of large doses of vitamin A and recovery from the measles. It has been an established fact for well over fifty years that children who are vitamin A deficient have a much harder time recovering from infectious diseases. These researchers found that if children with severe measles were given vitamin A in large doses (400,000 IU) starting during the first five days of the illness, the risk of complications is halved compared with their incidence in children given sugar pills instead. The dosage used was massive compared to the usual recommended daily allowance, but most of the children in the South African study were vitamin A deficient to begin with. The final recommendation of the study was that all children seriously ill with measles be treated with large doses of vitamin A. Well-nourished children with mild measles may not need massive doses of vitamin A, but should be given their usual vitamins regularly every day throughout the illness.

* * *

Foods with heavy, waxy coatings have been treated with mixtures of shellacs, paraffins, palm oil coatings, or synthetic resins—the same ingredients used to polish floors or cars. This wax spray is applied to apples, avocados, bell peppers, cantaloupes, cucumbers, eggplants, grapefruits, limes, lemons, and melons—just to name a few. A pound of wax coats 160,000 pieces of produce and reduces the moisture loss of food by 30-40%. The waxes in and of themselves are not a health hazard, however, they may trap pesticides, insecticides, and fungicides sprayed on plants during the growing season.

* * *

The International Banana Association has a helpful hint for banana peels—the inside of a banana peel makes an excellent shoe polish.

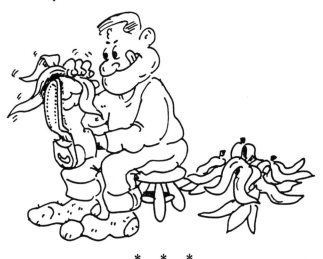

*   *   *

BODY TRIVIA
2

I n terms of light bulbs, the resting human gives off as much heat as a 150-watt bulb.

*   *   *

Gums are renewed every one to two weeks.

*   *   *

If it were possible to drain all of the water from a 72.6 kg (160 lb.) man, his dehydrated body would weigh a mere 29 kg or 64 pounds. Of that weight only 19 pounds are bone.

Speaking of bones, the only bone in the body that has no known function is the coccyx—man's vestigial tail.

*   *   *

The pressure in the aorta is such that if the aorta were opened, blood would spout a column six feet high.

*   *   *

The heart does enough work each day to lift the body a mile straight up in the air.

*   *   *

Tears drain down into the throat even when the body is hanging upside down.

* * *

A man snoozing in a hammock may absorb only ½ pint of oxygen per minute. However, a runner trying to break the world's record in the mile, may soak up more than five quarts of oxygen in the same period.

* * *

There are approximately 2.5 million nephrons to do the dirty work of excreting waste products via the kidneys. If all of the tubules 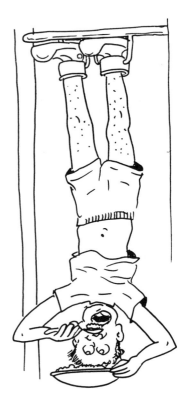 of the nephrons were stretched out, they would stretch for approximately 50 miles (80km). No wonder our kidneys can filter 180 liters per day and reabsorb 99% of that which is filtered.

* * *

Over a lifetime, a normal human heart will pump enough blood to fill 13 supertankers, each with a capacity of one million barrels.

* * *

Sitting perfectly still you shed more than a million flakes of skin every hour.

* * *

Each individual is so unique that the odds against duplication by the same parents are about 144 billion to one.

*   *   *

Well, here's an anthropological gem that will surely result in many sleepless nights. Our teeth are getting smaller. Yes, and we can blame this on the fact that we are cooking our own food. Teeth have shrunk in size by about 50% over the last 100,000 years. Don't worry, you won't wake up tomorrow with shorter teeth. They are shrinking, but only at the rate of 1% per 1,000 years.

*   *   *

Platelets are named after their resemblance to tiny plates. You know, like baby pigs are named after resemblance to their big pig parents—piglets.

*   *   *

As of May, 1989 it was estimated that Americans lugged around 1.5 billion extra pounds.

*   *   *

Your average pig squeals at 108 decibels, and the average chain saw hums along at 105 decibels. Your husband snores at 80 decibels—unless he's a pig.

Nearly one-half of average American adults snore occasionally. However, men who snore outnumber women 30 to 1.

The level in decibels of the loudest recorded snore is 87.5. This is the average decibel level of an alarm clock.

*   *   *

The human body is made up of 100 trillion cells. The human ovum is 1000 times bigger than any other cell in the body.

*   *   *

Why is it that women are plagued with the propensity to cry more often than men? It's probably due to hormones, and not social conditioning. The hormone believed to be responsible for this annoying phenomenon is prolactin. Prolactin is found in the tears of both sexes; however, women have 60% more prolactin in their blood than men. 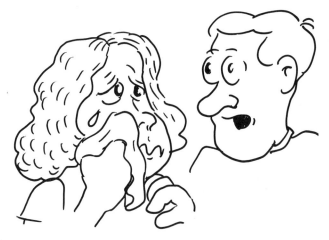 Before puberty, boys and girls have equal amounts of prolactin in their bloodstream and cry equally as often.

*   *   *

The human hand has 1,300 nerve endings per square inch.

*   *   *

The typical human cell, containing 50,000 genes made of an estimated 3 billion base pairs, takes about 7 hours to make one copy of all of its genes.

*   *   *

The brain undergoes 100,000 chemical reactions per second.

* * *

Here is a question that perhaps many of you have thought about but have never had the courage to ask. Why are yawns contagious? Is this not a query of importance that has mystified you for years? Has it kept you awake at night pondering the mechanism of transmission from one person to another? 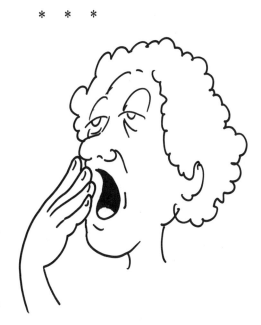 Why is it that when one even thinks of a yawn, it happens? Are you yawning now?

The answers to the above questions may be found in this newest study. Many of us might like to try out the findings. We know that yawns increase before bedtime and right after you wake up. We also know that we yawn when we're bored and that yawns are contagious. However, we don't know what triggers a yawn. Is it a response to decreased O_2 or increased CO_2? Most researchers think that it is not. Breathing and yawning are probably triggered by different internal states and are probably controlled by separate mechanisms. Breathing can be satisfactorily performed through either the nose or the mouth; however, researchers have reported that subjects find it very difficult if not impossible to perform a satisfying yawn with their mouth taped shut. And, oral inhalation by itself will not produce a satisfactory yawn unless the jaw is free to move. In other words, subjects attempting a yawn with clenched teeth often reported an unpleasant sensation of being stuck in mid-yawn—try it.

Yawning isn't always a sign of boredom. Perhaps you are related to a species of penguins, the Adelie penguins to be exact. In their world, the yawn is an erotic display.

* * *

Another tidbit on a bodily function. Did you know that it was theoretically impossible to burp in space? You need gravity to burp, and, of course, space has zero gravity.

* * *

Remember how they told you in General Chemistry 101 that the human body was only worth a few pennies in the chemical sense? They lied. A 154-pound human body contains $525 in cholesterol; $739.50 in fibrinogen; $2,500 in hemoglobin; $4,819.50 in albumin; $30,600 each in prothrombin and IgG; and $100,000 in myoglobin. The grand total comes to $169,834.00. But where do you go to cash in your chemicals?

* * *

The warmer an individual is, the longer he or she will sleep. Subjects who fell asleep when body temperatures were at their lowest point of their daily cycle slept 7.8 hours, while those who fell asleep during their highest daily temperature level averaged 14.4 hours of sleep.

* * *

MEDICAL MINUTIAE

Estimates indicate that there are approximately 650,000 microorganisms per square inch of human skin. In fact, there are more of these tiny critters on each of us than there are people in the world.

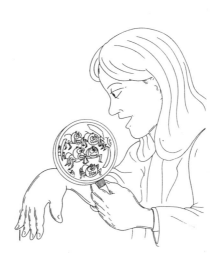

*   *   *

Did you know that if you just sat around and did NOTHING for 24 hours that you would burn approximately 1,700 calories? And no two people burn the same amount of calories even if they are both sitting and doing zero. National Institute of Health metabolism researchers studied 177 individuals who volunteered to live in a "respiratory chamber" that measures how much energy an individual expends in a 24-hour time period. Energy output was measured by monitoring oxygen consumption and CO_2 liberation. Radar guns and motion detectors were worn on the wrists to keep a record of the amount of fidgeting, such as toe tapping, finger drumming, and other such nervous movements were performed in the 24-hour period. The results of the study demonstrated that the variation among the volunteers ranged from 100 calories expended to 800 calories expended. Slim women fidget more than obese women, but the same pattern was not found in men. Within 27 families studied, brothers and sisters shared the fidgeting tendency.

*   *   *

Do you really want to know what cellulite is? Cellulite is a normal dimpling of the skin over such fatty areas as the hips and thighs. The pattern seems to have a genetic predisposition; however, the cellulite gene has not yet been isolated. (Once isolated let's hope that they can find a way to delete it once and for all. This will probably be one area of recombinant DNA research that will not receive any negative publicity, marches on Washington, or "the right to cellulite" groups.) When cellulite pops up, it's due to the dimpling of the skin caused by fat deposits that build up between the walls of connective tissue. As a person gains weight, the fat cells bulge upward from these confined spaces, pushing the skin into a pattern of bumps and puckers. The only way to remove cellulite is to remove fat through diet and exercise, in some cases through liposuction, and in other cases, dynamite.

*   *   *

Only 10% of the U.S. population is left-handed. However, more than half of the babies born two months prematurely are left-handed.

*   *   *

The recent results of a small research study from SUNY at Stonybrook found that left-handed individuals may be more sensitive to drugs that affect neurological functioning. The researchers gave 56 male college students 15 psychoactive drugs, one at a time, of course, and monitored the neuronal response after each drug. The most significant increases in brain activity occurred in left-handed individuals. Half of the left-handers ranked in the top 10% of drug-induced activity. The mildest responses to all drugs occurred in right-handers. When researchers tested placebos, they found no differences between the two groups. What does this study imply? Well, first of all, since the group was so small, it would have to be reproduced on a much larger scale for the results to have significance. However, a few implications may be surmised. Perhaps left-handed individuals need smaller doses of psychoactive drugs for long-term therapy. They may also be more sensitive to imbalances in the body's own drugs, which may explain why left-handers have more migraine headaches, seizure disorders, and learning disabilities.

* * *

The prevalence of obesity among 12 to 17 year olds increased by 2% with each hour of television viewed. Next to prior obesity, television viewing was found to be the most significant predictor of obesity in adolescence.

* * *

A study of highway rest stops in Washington State revealed that males averaged 45 seconds in the rest room, whereas

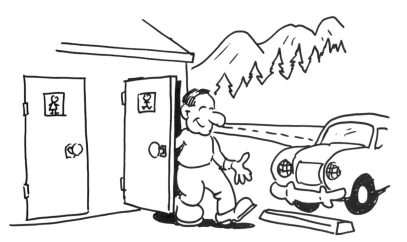

females averaged 79 seconds. The female engineering student researching this vital issue concluded that the 50:50 ratio between women's and men's toilet facilities in public rest rooms around the country was unfair.

*   *   *

The federal government spends an average of $19,100 every time the average American's heart beats. The interest on the national debt accumulates at the rate of $190,000 per minute.

And speaking of heartbeats, this is a good one for you. Some researchers theorize that each of us are pre-programmed to have only a certain number of heartbeats per lifetime. Which means, of course, that the faster you use them up, like exercising, the quicker you use up your allotment. (WOW, is this fuel for those folks who hate to exercise!)

Now don't burn your NIKE Airs so fast. Another physician whipped out his calculator and did some fancy figuring and found the following interesting facts: He assumed that the average non-jogging human has a resting heart rate of 72 beats per minute, and an average life span of 75 years. This works out to 2.832 billion beats per lifetime. In comparison, the conditioned runner who averages 45 minutes per day, 4-5 times per week from age 20-60 has a resting heart rate of 55. His exercise-induced heart rate is 180 beats per minute. Calculations show that he would run out of heartbeats by the age of 94, almost 20 years after the non-exercising counterpart.

*   *   *

For those of you who love those high-heeled pumps, head to your friendly orthopedist or chiropractor. Wearing high heels on a daily basis can lead to extreme curvature of the spine, lower back pain, permanent shortening of the Achilles tendon, and enlarged, displaced calf muscles. Not only that, but you walk funny. Feet clad in high-heeled shoes have a difficult time initiating locomotion. Normally the foot propels the leg by opening the angle between the toe and the bottom of the leg. With high-heels the angle is already open; therefore, it's hard to get-a-goin'; hence, you have difficulty walking.

Feet have grown progressively larger over the last few centuries. The average shoe size of soldiers in the Revolutionary War was 6C; in WWII it was 8D; and in 1984 it was 9½D.

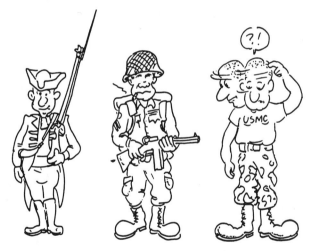

One more foot fact—the difference between shoe sizes is exactly 1 barleycorn or 1/3 of an inch. In other words, a size 7 is 1/3 of an inch longer than a size 6. A size 9 is exactly one inch longer than a size 6.

*　　*　　*

One out of every eleven American women will develop breast cancer in her lifetime. Some studies have indicated that having an increased number of children may decrease the risk of having breast cancer. Therefore the National Institute of Health performed one of its classic studies on dairy cows to see if there was any relationship between their breeding habits and the development of mammary cancer. They found that in those dairy cows that bred annually, there was udderly no mammary cancer. The moral of the story is to breed annually!

* * *

The largest newborn of record was a 24-pound 4-ounce boy in Turkey. The smallest newborn to survive was a 10-ounce female born in the U.S. in 1938. And speaking of babies, a Russian peasant woman gave birth to 69 children: 14 sets of twins, 7 sets of triplets, and 4 sets of quadruplets!

* * *

Sodium bicarb (i.e., Arm & Hammer baking soda) should not be taken on a full stomach. Case in point: a young gentleman consumed two margaritas, one order of Nachos, and a large Mexican combination plate for dinner. Upon arriving at home, he took ½ teaspoon of baking soda in water and within one minute experienced severe abdominal pain. Emergency surgery revealed a ruptured stomach. It was assumed that once the sodium bicarb hit the hydrochloric acid in the stomach, the combination of the two produced a carbon dioxide gas that was unable to exit the stomach, HENCE, THE EXPLOSION.

* * *

Approximately one to one and a half liters of saliva are secreted by our salivary glands each day. Most of this saliva is secreted during the day, with very little of it secreted at night. The bacteria that reside in our mouth know this important fact and, being the opportunists that they are, they divide more rapidly when we are asleep. And just to let you know that they have been quite busy during the night, they leave a nice film covering your teeth as well as a healthy dose of bad breath.

* * *

Peak smelling ability occurs between the ages of 30-50 and declines steadily afterwards. Women have a much keener sense of smell than men as well as better tasting abilities.

Estrogen gives females a greater sense of smell than males. A female can detect musk, the scent associated with male bodies, better than any other odor. When estrogen levels peak during ovulation, a woman's smell is most acute and can detect musk 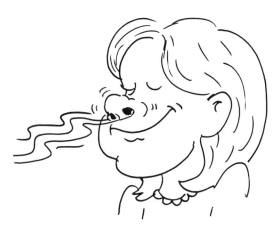 100-100,000 times more keenly than during menstruation.

* * *

Do you have or do you know anyone with uncontrollable hiccups? Here are two possible causes and remedies. Look carefully into the ear canal for a small foreign object that may be irritating the drum. Two cases reported to the *New England Journal of Medicine* found a bit of hair pressing against the tympanic membrane and the other reported a small ant. When the foreign items were removed, the patients recovered totally. Another case of intractable hiccups involved a 75-year-old woman. She had a 35-year history of hiccups until she developed Parkinson's disease and was treated with the drug Amantidine (Symmetrel). Her hiccups cleared immediately after the amantidine was started. When the amantidine was discontinued, her hiccups resumed in full force. So, keep this drug in mind if you ever happen upon someone with intractable hiccups.

*   *   *

Intractable sneezing has also been reported in the literature. One 11-year-old girl was admitted to the University of New Mexico Hospital after sneezing 20 times per minute for three weeks. One 17-year-old female had a history of continuous sneezing for 154 days. Still another woman was found to have sneezed for 3 years at a rate of 25 per minute.

Since we mentioned the sneeze, it was once thought that a healthy sneeze served to cleanse the brain. Hippocrates, in all of his infinite wisdom, considered the sneeze as a dangerous sign of lung disease but also curative for some cases of hiccups.

Approximately 20 percent of the population sneeze when they walk out into the light or look at a bright light. This is known as the photic sneeze reflex and has been known for centuries. The exact physiologic mechanism for this effect is unknown; however, it is believed to be due to intricate connections in the visual pathways that activate the receptors in the respiratory system. Research suggests that the photic sneeze is an inherited trait and is passed in an autosomal dominant pattern. They have even given this genetic predisposition a clever name with the acronym ACHOO— auto-somal dominant compelling helio-ophthalmic outburst syndrome—whatever that means. It's hypothesized that there is a selective advantage to being an overly sensitive sneezer. Arctic and cold climate populations are constantly exposed to respiratory tract infections but the frequent sneezes in the group have less infections and get sick less often. They forcefully expel the germs before the germs have a chance to get into the body.

Just how forceful is a sneeze? The velocity of the sneeze is approximately 100 MPH, just in case you were wondering. During a normal exhale the velocity is 15 MPH. Sneeze particles are propelled 1½ to 6 feet (approximately 100 feet per second). During the first few minutes after a sneeze the bacterial count in the immediate vicinity of the room increases by 500 per cubic millimeters.

* * *

Since we have talked about sneezes and hiccups, let's give a few moments to the eyeblink reflex. In the not so distant past, one method of torture was to snip off the eyelids. Victims eventually went blind as the cornea dried up and clouded over.

Obviously, the eyeblink is a protective reflex that preserves and protects the eye.

- Infants under the age of two months blink once a minute.
- Children blink about six times per minute.
- Dogs and cats blink about two times per minute.

- By the age of 20, humans blink approximately 24 times per minute.

When we get bored or tired we blink more frequently. For example, after driving an hour on a long stretch of boring highway, we blink over 40 times per minute. We also blink more often when we are angry or when we are talking to the boss, or when we are embarrassed. We decrease our blinking when reading; however, we often blink each time we come to a period at the end of the sentence. Blink. The more difficult the text, the less frequently we blink.

*   *   *

Researchers have observed that myopia (nearsightedness) is more often seen among people with high intelligence, high educational levels, and high academic achievement. Physicians studied 158,000 men age 17-19 years and found a strong association between the prevalence of myopia and both intelligence and schooling.

Verbally- and mathematically-gifted children are more likely than children of average ability to be left-handed, nearsighted, and suffering from allergies. Researchers suggest that these variables may be biological correlates of intelligence. It would be interesting to find out if the researchers were lefties, wore thick bifocals, and took mega doses of anti-histamines, eh?

*   *   *

How do we produce sounds? Our vocal cords, which are thick tough folds of connective tissue and ligament, produce sounds by vibrating as exhaled air puffs through them. The vibrations are extremely rapid—125 cycles per second in men, 200 cycles per second in women. Differences in length and thickness of vocal folds largely account for the contrast in frequency, which our ears perceive as pitch. In men, the folds are typically 7/8" to 1¼" long. In women, they're ¼" shorter on the average and half as thick. Consequently men have lower voices.

*   *   *

Are you a short duration sleeper or do you like to sleep for days? One group of investigators reported that if you are a short duration sleeper you are more active in attempting to master your life than the long-duration sleepers who take a more fatalistic approach.

*   *   *

U.S. babies dirty 18 billion disposable diapers per year. Only 15% of all diapers used per year are washed and recycled. This preference for disposables adds an extra 550 bucks per year to your baby budget.

*   *   *

The number of laughs an average person has in one day is 15.

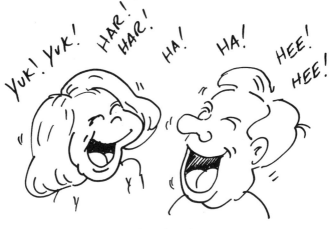

*   *   *

The average number of dreams per year is 1,460.

*   *   *

It takes approximately 20 seconds for a drop of blood to make it through the systemic circulation.

*   *   *

The ability to taste diminishes with age. If you place a small electrical stimulus with a metallic taste on the tongue, 82% of individuals between the ages of 20-30 will perceive it, whereas only 16% over the age of 52 will perceive it.

A 12-year-old child has approximately 248 lingual papillae (taste buds); a 75-year-old has only 88. Is it any wonder that the elderly have a decreased interest in food?

*   *   *

You can expect to fall or trip on stairs once every 72,000 times that you use them. Do we actually use stairs that much? One researcher from Georgia Tech calls stairs the most dangerous consumer product after automobiles. This same researcher also stated that the U.S. has between 1.8 and 2.6 million accidents involving stairs per year. And just in case you're thinking about your next stair mishap (in other words, are you on your 71,999th step ready to hit 72,000?) just remember that more people fall UP the stairs than down the stairs. Do you think that Ralph Nader will go after stairs next?

*   *   *

The June 18, 1988 *British Medical Journal* published an interesting report on kids with food allergies. Grade school kids who had finicky eating habits and food allergies were more than a half inch shorter than their classmates. The height differences increased with the number of foods a child could not eat. If the child reported three or more food allergies, he or she tended to be more than an inch and a half shorter than average.

*   *   *

Ladies, are you tired of your Maidenform losing its shape, its lift, its zip-a-dee-do-dah? Nippon Zeon, a manufacturer of plastics and synthetic rubber, has created the first bra with a memory. Can you stand it? Yes, my friends, your new cross-your-heart Nippon Zeon will regain its lift, its shape, its zip-a-dee-do-dah when you drop it into hot water—that's all it takes to restore it's original form.

*   *   *

Many feminist writers have rebelled against our sexist English language. They have vowed to change the "no-MEN-clature" not only in everyday language, such as mail person and womyn, but also in the medical field. Keeping all of these important changes in mind I came across this little ditty:

> I wonder if our new estate
> will alter nature's laws
> Will wopersons personstruate
> until personopause?

*   *   *

If you work night shifts you are 30% more prone to have accidents at work than those who work days, especially if the shift worker changes shifts frequently. Changing shifts not only causes sleep disturbances but it also changes the times of day at which certain regulatory hormones such as epinephrine and thyroid hormone are most abundant. Hormone production cannot change as quickly—in fact it can only adjust its production by about one hour per 24-hour period. For workers who change shifts, it is suggested that the rotation last at least two weeks. In addition, certain drugs utilized in the treatment of diabetes mellitus, hypertension, seizure disorders, and asthma also interact with hormonal production and may cause increased problems in those individuals doing shift work. It is recommended that individuals taking medications for any of the aforementioned disorders avoid working shifts.

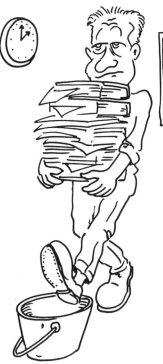

*   *   *

Is there life after death? Who knows? However, we do know that there is brain wave activity after death. A researcher reported that dead brains continued to send out signals for an average of 37 hours. The longest brain activity was 168 hours or 7 days.

*   *   *

"Long in the tooth" is a slang term for getting older, but what does it really mean? Two mechanisms are responsible for older people growing "long in the tooth." First of all, bone mineral content is lost with aging due to osteoporosis and periodontal disease, and the maxilla and mandible are not exceptions. This loss causes the gum tissue to retract from the teeth. In addition, our gums tend to shrink with age and this also contributes to the "long in the tooth."

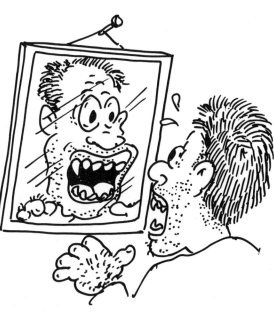

*   *   *

Hitachi Metals in Japan has developed a method of attaching false teeth by magnet to a stainless steel plate embedded in the top of the mouth. What, pray tell, might happen if you're sipping soup? Will the metal spoon attach mercilessly to the upper plate? What if two people with magnetic mouths kiss? Can you imagine the walls of a magnetic resonance facility, decorated with human sculptures attached to the walls by their gums?

*   *   *

After age 63, a woman's walking pace slows by 12.3% per decade, whereas the average man slows his gait by 16.1%. From age 19-62, there is a 1-2% decline per decade in the normal walking speed of men and women alike. In addition, individuals over age 63 take shorter steps than those in the 19-62 age group.

* * *

Suffering from unsightly cracked heels? You're not alone—another 17,999,999 Americans are suffering with you. The best remedy is to soak your feet in warm water for 20 minutes, gently rub a pumice stone over the affected area to remove some of the dead skin, and pat dry. Then apply Dr. Scholls *Cracked Heel Relief Cream*—a guaranteed remedy.

* * *

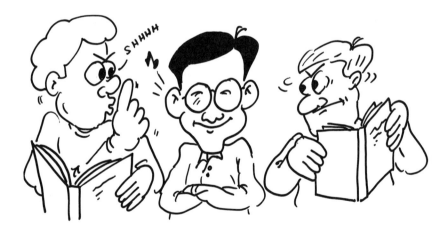

A 25-year-old Japanese patient was admitted to the hospital with a continuous high pitched tone coming out of his right ear. He couldn't hear it, but all of those around him could. As usual, in medicine, everything must have a name.

His condition was referred to as spontaneous otoacoustic emission, etiology unknown. The treatment consisted of anesthetizing the eardrum, and the noise abated.

* * *

A question that has nagged many of us for years—just what is done with all of the circumicised foreskin? Circumcised foreskins have been shown to have clinical use—a Boston University dermatologist is growing the tissue in a special culture medium that increases the surface area of the foreskin up to 10,000 times. The resulting translucent material is attached to a gauze pad and then placed on a wound. The young cells release a multitude of growth factors that stimulate the aging cells to begin growing and repairing the damaged tissue.

Circumcised foreskin is also being used to test make-up instead of using animal skin.

* * *

During the usual night's sleep, the body shifts position between 40 and 70 times. The purpose of this flipping and flopping is to maintain a healthy circulation and muscle tone.

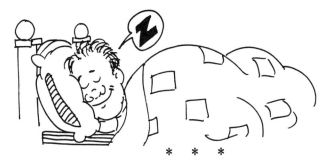

* * *

Talk about a quick-thinking fast-acting father—an Alaskan Eskimo father freed his son's tongue that was frozen to a handrail by urinating on it. Usually, warm water is more acceptable treatment, but access to warm, running water may be limited in many situations, especially in an Eskimo village in Alaska. (letter—*New England Journal of Medicine.*)

*   *   *

Why do people who live together long enough start to look alike? Is it diet? Is it in the water? No, researchers at the University of Michigan attribute the resemblance to shared similar emotional experiences over the years. Therefore they tend to reflect each others facial expressions in what is referred to as "repeated empathic mimicry". The theory is that facial expressions can change the lines and contour of the face over time, and similar patterns of facial expressions will sculpt similar faces. An additional implication of this theory is that kin resemblance may not strictly be a matter of genetics, but "repeated empathic mimicry" may also play a role here.

*   *   *

How about a pocket breath-o-lyzer? A gadget that electrically senses levels of methyl mercaptan, the primary ingredient that causes halitosis, has been developed for personal use. Three blinking lights let you know whether you are kissable, borderline, or completely repulsive.

*   *   *

A psychologist from Rennsalaer Polytechnical Institute studied the reaction of individuals to various physical characteristics of strangers. Here are two of the findings: 1) facial hair (especially a beard) makes a man seem older, less attractive and less sociable as compared to his clean-shaven counterparts; 2) balding men were perceived as smarter, a little older, and more mature. In addition, the presence of cranial hair had no effect on how the viewer rated relative attractiveness.

* * *

Speaking of facial hair, another astounding piece of research has emerged from the Sackler School of Medicine , Tel-Aviv University, Israel. Non-Ashkenazi Jewish men who have mustaches on the lower part of their upper lip have an unusually high rate of peptic ulcer disease and dyspepsia. The researcher speculated that men who trim their mustaches into a narrow line are obsessive, perfectionist extroverts— personality traits that have always been linked to excessive hydrochloric acid production in the upper GI tract. Over 100 non-Ashkenazi Jews, aged 18-79, who had half mustaches, were compared to 107 controls, most of whom had full mustaches. Almost three times as many men in the half-mustached group had proven ulcer disease and about twice as many had dyspepsin, compared to the controls.

And yet another hairy note: A neuropsychiatrist at UC-Irvine has been studying the chemical elements of hair samples from violent criminals in California state prisons and comparing the amounts to non-criminals. The most significant finding was that the violent criminals had five times as much manganese in their hair. The researcher is now looking for a link between high levels of manganese, brain lesions, and violent behavior. Whether manganese is a marker or a direct cause of violent behavior is not known; however, the manganese is significantly elevated and does show some type of abnormal metabolism in this group.

* * *

Two cell types have been shown to have specific receptors for THC (tetrahydrocannabinol) the active ingredient in marijuana. When THC combines with neurons, mood elevation ensues, colors become brighter, munchies become tastier, and a dried floral arrangement can be the focus of intense discussion for hours. Studies on the effects of marijuana on fertilization, performed on the sea urchin, have found THC receptors are also present on their sperm. When a sea urchin's sperm were sprayed with THC, the rate of fertilization declined by 99.5% most likely due to the THC blocking the "docking" site of the sperm onto the egg. Since the sea urchin belongs to a phylum that includes vertebrates like those of us reading this, it is believed that we have a common ancestor—at least we did 600-800 million years ago. Therefore, the THC receptor must be at least that old. For it to have been around for all these years it must have some function of major importance.

* * *

One way to check the temperature when you're outdoors is to inhale rapidly. If you feel the moisture in your nostrils begin to freeze, it is 10° F or colder.

* * *

Male pattern baldness, a receding hairline coupled with a bald spot on the crown of the head, tends to correlate with hypertension and hypercholesterolemia. A study of 872 Italian males showed that the connection between baldness and cardiovascular risk was independent of age, body fat, and diet. The underlying cause is most likely hormonal. High levels of testosterone have been linked to male pattern baldness and may be responsible for higher cholesterol levels and blood pressure levels as well.

* * *

Ever heard of hereditary localized pruritus? Well, it's an itchy spot that runs in families. For example, that hard-to-reach area between the scapula may be just as itchy in you as it is in your mom. Dermatologists hypothesize that it's caused by a hereditary susceptibility to mild sensory nerve injury, which in turn stimulates the itching sensation.

* * *

The *International Journal of Dermatology* (December 1988) reports that severe itching of the nose can be a sign of a brain tumor or heart disease. That interesting tidbit deserves more of an explanation—I'll keep you posted as I delve into the pathophysiology.

* * *

Problems with foot odor? Most problems with foot odor stem from the combination of excessive sweating and the overgrowth of bacteria on the feet. Here are three remedies that you might want to try: 1) an aqueous solution of aluminum chlorhydrate dispersed in isopropyl alcohol, sprayed on the feet daily to reduce perspiration, 2) chlorhexidine gluconate (Hibiclens) every day as a bactericidal agent, or 3) the use of Clindamycin (Cleocin), an antibiotic, daily.

* * *

Lightning is considered to be quite an occupational hazard for church bell ringers. In the Middle Ages it was a common practice to ring church bells to disperse thunder. This practice was not very successful for obvious reasons; however, the success rate of a lightning bolt hitting a bell tower was quite high. When lightning struck a bell tower it most often took the bell ringer with it.

Edwin Robinson of Falmouth, Maine had been blind for 9 years when he was struck by lightning in 1980. The bolt knocked him out; however, when he came to he was able to see again. The postulated mechanism was the electrical shock rewiring the visual circuits.

*   *   *

Lawyers are 3.6 times more likely to suffer depression than people in other fields. Secretaries and school counselors ranked next.

*   *   *

Die-hard runners are at high risk for the development of gall stones. This is presumably a consequence of chronic intravascular hemolysis from red blood cell damage from running. Also these individuals are at risk for iron-deficiency anemia, basically for the same reason. The constant pounding on the pavement results in microscopic bleeding into the tissues. This in turn causes a loss of iron and a resultant iron-deficiency anemia.

*   *   *

The number of sperm cells as well as the motility of sperm cells are decreased for up to six weeks after a one hour session in the hot tub. A 102.4° temperature for one hour can cause immediate damage to sperm. Most health clubs keep their hot tubs at 104°F. Fertility is at its lowest four weeks after the hot tub session, when sperm that were immature upon bathing are finally matured. Is this permanent? Nope. The average life span of a sperm is 75 days, so all damaged sperm are replaced within that time—provided of course, there hasn't been another session in the hot tub.

*   *   *

The ovary is the most precisely and quantitatively doomed organ in the human body. In other words, it is preprogrammed to degenerate at a certain rate, regardless of your race, color, or religious background. At 5 months gestation, the female ovaries contain approximately 7 million eggs; however, in the following 4 months, 6.6 million eggs degenerate. At birth, each ovary contains 200,000 eggs, for a total of 400,000. That of course means that we have 400,000 periods to look forward to in a lifetime, but in actuality, the average American female has only 460 normal periods in a lifetime. Back to the original story. The eggs continue to degenerate as scheduled, so that a 30-year-old female has only 100,000 eggs. By age 50, we have exactly 3 eggs left. Count 'em: 3. (By the way, these eggs might be 50 years old, but they are still "lookin' for love." A woman can become pregnant at 50—she needs only one egg to do so). Once all of our eggs are depleted, we enter "the menopause."

So then, what about the sperm? Since women have all the eggs they're ever going to get at birth, do men have all the sperm they're going to get at birth? No, men produce sperm until the day they die. The only major difference between the sperm of a 20-year-old versus a 70-year-old is how fast the sperm can swim. The sperm from a 20-year-old can find an egg in approximately 50 minutes; whereas it takes 2½ days for the the sperm of a 70-year-old to reach its goal. Sperm only live 2½ days, so when they reach their goal, the egg, they die.

*   *   *

A study from a London hospital found that two out of every five nurses harbored disease-causing bacteria on the skin under their rings.

Even your toothbrush isn't safe...toothbrushes harbor infectious bacteria and fungi. They should be replaced at the start of any respiratory infection and replaced again when you recover from the illness.

*   *   *

Researchers at the University of California at San Francisco have found that women, on average, tolerate body temperatures about one degree high than men before they start to perspire. However, once they start, women sweat as much, on average, as do men.

*   *   *

The amount of stress placed on the heart during intercourse with one's usual partner is no greater than walking five level blocks or climbing two flights of stairs. In other words, the burden on the heart is negligible. Most physicians feel that post-heart attack patients can resume sexual intercourse in approximately 6 weeks, but most patients don't for an average of 13.6 weeks. The major reason given by the patients is fear of another heart attack due to the exertion.

Research however, has shown that this fear is not warranted. The overall death rate during intercourse is less than 1% of the total cardiac deaths. Interestingly enough greater than 90% of this small number are reported in individuals participating in sexual activity with someone other than their regular partner. (Hmmmm) One other contributing factor was the over-consumption of food or drink prior to the endeavor.

*   *   *

The proportion of women giving birth for the first time after age 35 increased 350% between 1980 and 1990, with second births over age 40 rising by the same amount.

* * *

The common cups used in communion may be spreading common bacteria. Researchers reporting in the *Annals of Internal Medicine* found bacteria on 12 of the 16 cups tested. Some of the organisms are "notorious" for causing disease.

* * *

Myocardial infarctions are highest following the holidays: 28% higher the day after Easter, 17% higher on July 5, and 16% higher on January 2. Also, men are 21% more likely to suffer an MI on their birthdays. Why? Increased emotional stress and over indulgence in food, alcohol, and nicotine. (Wilson A. Robert Wood Johnson Medical School, Dept. of Epidemiology, New Brunswick, NJ)

* * *

CRITTERS & BUGGERS
3

F orty percent of all pets are overweight.

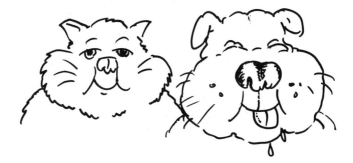

* * *

The oldest known mammal with syphilis was turned up in none other than Fulton County, Indiana last year. The victim was "short-faced bear" (an extinct species) who was stricken some 11,500 years ago with a syphilis-like disease. The manner in which he contracted the disease is not known—he could have devoured an infected human; however, the earliest human case of syphilis is only 5,000 years old.

* * *

That little vermin, the flea, can leap six inches up in the air and covers as much as two feet in a single bound. Weight for weight this would be the equivalent of man leaping one-fourth of a mile in a single bound.

Flea entomologists have clocked the rat flea jumping 30,000 times without stopping. One species of fleas can accelerate 50 times faster than the space shuttle. Some fleas

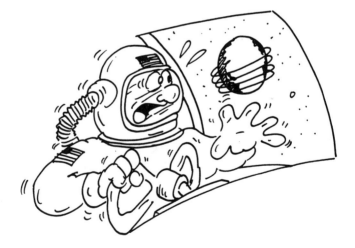

can live for months without a bite to eat, and still others can survive being placed in a freezer for one year. We should marvel at these little vermin. Unfortunately they also carry illness in the form of the plague, and they have caused more deaths than all wars ever fought.

* * *

Cats spend about 75% of their day snoozing. Gorillas and possums sleep 80% of the time, and woodchucks spend 92% of the time sawin' those zzzzz's. Contrary to the snoozin' group, sharks and the albatross hardly sleep at all, and the most unusual sleeping habits belong to the dolphin—it sleeps one hemisphere of the brain at a time.

* * *

The veins of an elephant ear form a pattern as unique as the human fingerprint.

* * *

In this era that places so much emphasis on athletic prowess we tend to forget that our athletic records appear rather paltry next to our counterparts in the animal world. For example, the human world record for the long jump is 29 feet 2.5 inches—a record that may never again be equaled in the human world. The Australian kangaroo scoffs at such a meager jump. The record kangaroo jump in Kangaroo Kingdom is 42 feet.

The human high jump record is 7 feet 10 inches; however, once again the Kangaroo has us beat—10 feet. Humans are pitiful when it comes to swimming. The human record for cruising through the water is 5.3 m.p.h. The penguin (which, of course, is actually a bird) moves through the water at 22

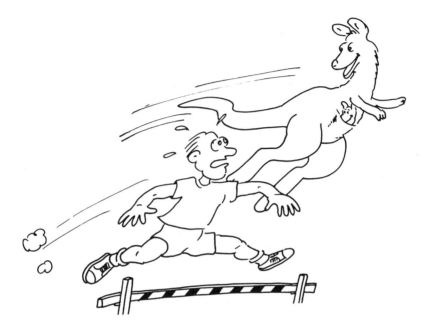

m.p.h. Humans can't even fall through the air with the greatest of speed. A free-falling human sky-diver can reach 185 m.p.h., but he will be promptly passed by the peregrine falcon which can plunge at speeds up to 275 m.p.h.

* * *

The development of the CAT scan relied on the pig as its research animal. Too bad it wasn't named as such.

* * *

Don't be offended when someone grunts and tells you that you eat like a pig. Pigs don't overeat. They produce a hormone, CCK or cholecystokinin, which transmits a message from the pork's belly to the pork's brain that says, "Stop pigging out."

Since this hormone acts as an appetite suppressant, pharmaceutical companies are already licking their chops over the possibilities for the human masses. Blocking the hormone could also prove to be beneficial to anorexics. When CCK is blocked in pigs, the animals will eat anything and everything.

More on pigs, eating, and the release of CCK...a report in the September 15, 1988 *New England Journal of Medicine* compares a group of women with bulimia with a group of women the same age and weight without bulimia. After eating a standard liquid meal, plasma levels of CCK and the subjective sense of satiety were both significantly lower in bulimics than in controls. This can mean one of two things, 1) it can reflect a causal role for impaired CCK release in bulimia, or 2) bulimia may lead to a secondary impairment of CCK release, which would then further enhance appetite and encourage binge eating.

* * *

OK, here's that answer to a question that has kept many of us awake at night. What does a bird use his or her wishbone for? Humanoids grab each end of the slippery little bone and make a wish, but it must be in the bird for a reason, correct? Well, each end of the wishbone is attached to one of the bird's two shoulders. Rapid compressions of the wishbone during flight squeezes air back and forth between the two lungs and between various sacs that serve to cool and lighten the bird's body. By squeezing and expanding these air sacs, the wishbone increases the amount of oxygen in the lungs; a big bonus during the high energy, high oxygen demanding exertions of flight.

* * *

Four hundred and fifteen babies are born every hour. In contrast, 2,000 dogs and 3,500 cats are born every hour.

*   *   *

Here's an interesting note: The February 1988 issue of *Pathophysiology Perspectives* was devoted to Lyme Disease, which, as you may remember, is caused by a little spirochete carried around on ticks which in turn are carried by dogs. A physician from Essex, Connecticut, where Lyme disease is endemic, noted that his Schnoodle (part Schnauzer/part Poodle) was "enjoying his usual excellent health until about two months ago when he developed a transient hind leg limp." His wife rushed the dog to the veterinarian who drew Lyme titres. The titres were strongly positive and oral tetracycline was prescribed. Of course, Schnoodle compliance with oral antibiotics has not been studied extensively; therefore, it's hard to ascertain how much of the prescribed antibiotic was taken. Two weeks later, the owner noted that the pooche's black nose seemed to be pointing to the left instead of straight ahead in the normal position. In addition, he was unable to close his left eye. The Schnoodle was exhibiting the classic signs of Lyme disease—the initial arthritis (with the limp), followed by the most common peripheral neuropathy, a facial nerve paralysis, or Bell's palsy.

*   *   *

A ten-gram hummingbird burns ten times as much oxygen per gram of body weight as the energetic human. To do this, the bird's heart beats about 1,440 times per minute compared to the heart of an exercising human that beats anywhere from 110-220.

*   *   *

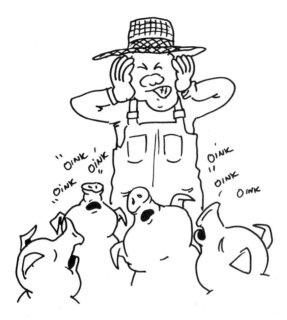

Back to Pigs. Pig farmers may have an occupational health hazard that they were previously unaware of—hearing damage. According to the British Department of Employment, the squeals of pigs at feeding time can reach a dangerous 108 decibels. (A chain saw produces 105 decibels in comparison). The agency cautioned farmers to wear ear muffs while slopping the hogs because even a 7.5 minute dose of multiple pig squeals can cause hearing damage...oink.

*   *   *

An allergist from Harvard Medical School has reported that up to 50% of the allergic individuals in the Boston area who are exposed to roaches will develop an allergic sensitivity to the pests. So, keep your nose out of the garbage, off the kitchen counter, and out from under the dining or kitchen table (the most popular places to catch the little monsters).

And speaking of roaches, for every one roach found, there are 800-2000 hiding. According to a team of cockroach specialists from the Agricultural Research Center in Gainesville, Florida, 97.5% of 1,000 low-income apartments were infested with a minimum of 160 roaches per dwelling (RPD), with an average of (you aren't going to believe this one) 33,600 roaches per dwelling, and up to 250,000 roaches per dwelling in the worst cases.

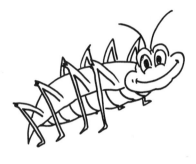

Unlike most insects, cockroaches have a relatively long life span. Three to four years is the norm for this group, and this has baffled researchers for decades. An answer may be forthcoming. It appears as if the roach has quite a sophisticated immune system, similar to that found in humans. Obviously it's not as sophisticated, but the two systems share important characteristics. In order for an immune system to work efficiently it has to have a memory. In other words, once you meet the pathogen, subsequent exposures will elicit an even stronger response. Roaches have developed the capacity to deal with repeated exposures to a multitude of environmental pathogens. A second similar characteristic is that female roaches have a much stronger and more sophisticated immune system than do male roaches. Baby roaches, the equivalent to our neonate, are immunoincompetant. Their immune systems have to learn from experience, as do ours. A third similar characteristic is the decline in immune function with aging. The three- to four-year-old roaches demonstrate an immune system that is waning in its ability to recognize and respond to foreign pathogens. One last similarity is that both roaches and humans produce a neutralizing protein to the offending agent. Ours is called IgA and theirs has not been characterized as yet. Suffice it to say, these prehistoric insects are not to be reviled, they are to be admired as a true masterpiece of the evolutionary process.

*   *   *

On to rats and a question we've all pondered: Why don't rats die of complications of atherosclerosis such as coronary artery disease? It appears as if they have specialized bacteria in their intestines that converts cholesterol to coprostanol, a

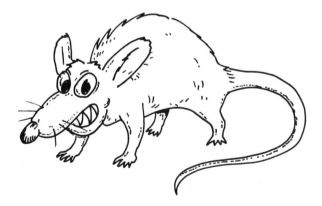

harmless metabolite that passes through the GI tract without being absorbed. Unfortunately these bacteria are virtually impossible to work with in the laboratory setting because they die when exposed to oxygen and they can only live on cultures of minced cow's brains. Yum!

The search was on for a similar bacteria that was easier to work with. A Ph.D. candidate from Iowa State University searched high and low (mostly low) in animal feces, river sludge, fetid ponds and in a sewage lagoon filled with run-off from a hog farm. The bacteria (s)he found is aptly referred to as *Eubacterium HL*, with the *HL* standing for hog lagoon. This study species lives on room air, lagoon air, any air, and can thrive in a lab on common soybean extracts. The good news is that when presented with cholesterol, they convert 90% of it to coprostanol. Researchers hope to characterize and mass produce the enzyme produced by the bacteria. This purified enzyme could possibly be sprinkled on food before we eat it or we could pack the enzyme into a capsule to break down the cholesterol in our GI tract.

* * *

Did you know that the healthy human liver weighs two to three pounds? Elsewhere in the animal world, the great white shark has a liver that comprises 20% of its total body weight. Therefore, an 800 lb. great white shark has a liver that weighs 160 pounds. Why? The shark must subsist for weeks and sometimes months on its fat reserves, and this just so happens to be where fat is stored.

* * *

We've used plants as sources of drugs for centuries. But now a new source is blossoming—using bugs for drugs. Of particular importance is the well-known diving beetle which produces corticosteroids. One such beetle can produce more steroid than what researchers used to squeeze out of the adrenal glands from hundreds of cows.

* * *

The part of a bloodhound's nose that does the smelling is 50 times larger and one million times more sensitive than a human nose.

*   *   *

More birds fall off fence posts and crash into picture windows in the spring than at any other time of the year. While traveling back to the northern climates during the spring, the birds munch on fruit that has been fermenting since the fall. This alcohol effect slows their reaction time and coordination rendering them unable to maintain their balance. Sound familiar?

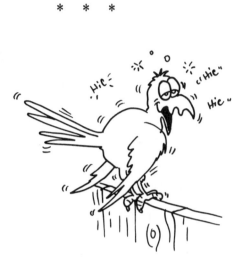

*   *   *

A fly has a lightning flash reflex and reaction time of less than one two hundredth of a second—10 times quicker than that of a fly swatter attached to a human hand.

*   *   *

The night owl (great-horned owl) has 14 vertebrae in its neck, giving it the unique ability to swirl its head through three-fourths of a complete circle. It needs this mobility because of the size of its eyes which are so large that there is no room in the head for the extraocular muscles that usually move the eyes.

*   *   *

Just in case you're in cahoots with a dairy farmer, the 43rd International Science and Engineering Fair in Nashville shed some light on cow's preferences for music. An eight-week study found that cows increased their production of milk by 6.2% if they listened to country music. Rock music only increased the output by 4.7%, and Mozart was a dismal failure—only a 1.6% increase with classical music. Now that's a kick in the dairy air.

*   *   *

The February 1, 1992 *Journal of Epidemiology* concluded that dogs with long noses are protected from the carcinogenic effects of passive smoke from their owners. An epidemiologist from Colorado State University sifted through the oncology records maintained by two veterinary hospitals in the Ft. Collins, Colorado area. He identified 51 dogs with lung cancer and 83 control dogs with various other types of malignancy. Tobacco smoke exposure was estimated by sending a questionnaire to the owners. A statistically significant link was found between exposure to passive smoke and lung cancer with short and medium-size muzzles. Dogs with long muzzles showed no excess of lung cancer while they resided with a smoking owner. Why? It would appear that the length of the nasal passage contributes to a filtering effect of the carcinogens in cigarette smoke.

*   *   *

Raw turkey breasts are being used to test the effectiveness of surgical gloves. Since turkey breasts have a texture very similar to human skin, researchers are operating on turkey breasts to determine how well the gloves block bacteria during operating techniques such as cutting, suturing, and stapling.

* * *

A new assay is being tested to determine the number of insect fragments in grain products. The current process is to do a gross inspection by spreading out grain kernels and eye-balling them for whole insects or insect fragments. To pick out the smaller segments, they cook up this elaborate concoction, shake it up, filter off what floats to the top, dry the extract, and look at it under the microscope. Just so you realize the complexity of the job, "It takes six months of training to become an insect-fragment counter," says Dr. Barrie Kitto, Mr. Insect-Fragment Counter, himself.

The new assay, researched by Dr. Kitto, measures myosin, a muscle protein present in insects at all life stages. When an extraction fluid is added to grain or foods containing the myosin, the mix turns green. The deeper the hue, the greater amount of myosin in the grain. Using a color meter, one can quantitate each reading.

Current federal standards allow 75 insect fragments per 50 grams of grain, but here's the clincher—fragment size. Whether it's three-fourths of a large maggot or just a measly fruit fly's wing tip is immaterial.

* * *

A study reported by Lee Siegel, AP science writer, published in the Kinsport, Tennessee local newspaper, has finally explained the etiology of global warming. Scientists who have been studying fossilized dinosaur dung have issued a consensus statement, the gist of which is: Dinosaur flatulence may have helped warm Earth's prehistoric climate. This prehistoric greenhouse effect was due to the copious amounts of methane produced when digesting their food via the fermenting process. This, of course, lends support to the $216,000 study on modern day global warming caused by or aggravated by belching cows, sheep, and other livestock that ferment their food. Who ever said that Congress was out of its mind when it approved the money to research the current patterns of livestock eructations?

*   *   *

And yet another use for pigs. Researchers from Purdue University are using the pig's small intestinal mucosa to make tissue grafts for replacing worn-out blood vessels, ligaments, and bladders. The Purdue team has transplanted the material into over 600 animals of various species without any signs of immune rejection. Since this material has an anti-coagulant property, it was first used to replace the aortae in dogs. Within two months the graft had been replaced by the dog's own blood vessel tissue, a phenomenon referred to as remodeling. A similar phenomenon occurred in the vena cava when this material was used. It has also been used to replace canine knee ligaments and Achilles tendons. Within a few weeks the pig mucosa became fully developed ligament and tendon tissue.

Another use is to inject the pig mucosa into the bladder to strengthen its muscles and reduce incontinence. Future plans include testing this material to promote wound healing when used as a skin graft.

*   *   *

Speaking of animal intestines, it takes the intestines from two cows to provide sufficient gut to make one tennis racket. Yes, I said cow intestines not cat gut. Cat gut is a misnomer that took hold over 200 years ago. At the time, sheep intestines were used to make violin strings. As the tale has it, the instrument sounded like a cat screeching, and this became the generic term for natural animal gut.

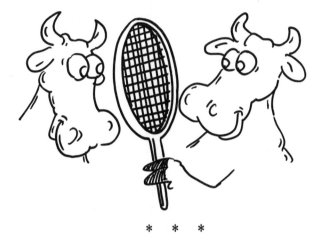

* * *

Can you believe that a cow needs about three pounds of water to make one pound of milk?

* * *

WHY NOT EAT INSECTS? is the title of a book written in 1885. It contains recipes for such scrumptious delicacies as slug soup, braised beef with caterpillars, boiled neck of mutton with none other than wireworm sauce, and gooseberry cream with sawflies. HUNGRY?

* * *

What's the best way to remove bugs from the ear canal? One old remedy is to put a drop of mineral oil in the ear canal.

Will this work? Doctors in the emergency room at Charity Hospital in New Orleans had a chance to perform the first scientifically controlled test of this bug-in-the-ear folk remedy. A patient entered the emergency room with two live roaches—one conveniently located in each ear. One ear received the drop of mineral oil, while the other received a squirt of lidocaine, a local anesthetic. The result: The lidocaine won. It caused the roach to seize, release it's grip on the ear canal, and fall out. The mineral oil simply suffocated the roach and the doctors had to probe the ear canal to remove it.

* * *

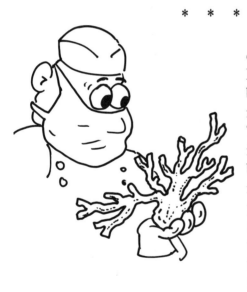

Certain species of coral from the South Pacific are being used by plastic surgeons to reconstruct jaw bones. This sea coral is nearly identical to human bone in terms of mineral content and porousness. In addition, it stimulates the body's natural bone tissue to infiltrate and strengthen the implant.

* * *

FUN FACTS FOR THE FECAL MINDED
4

O kay, here it is—the answer to why stools float when you eat a healthier diet (i.e., high fiber). They float because of trapped gas from colonic fermentation of non-digestible fiber. Therefore, it is much healthier to have stools that are "floaters" vs. "sinkers."

* * *

Flatus, as we all know, is the medical term for intestinal gas. There are actually individuals in this world who make a living studying the formation of flatus, or flatulence as it were. Would this group of researchers be called flatulentologists? Foods that produce gas are referred to as flatulogenic foods—beans, beans, and more beans, Brussels sprouts, raisins, apricots, celery, and onions, just to name a few. Are you plagued by the excess production of flatus? If so, you can make an appointment with your local flatulentologist for your very own flatulogram.

The elimination of flatulence is proportionate to the amount of gas formed. Under normal circumstances, the average American adult passes between 200-2000 ml of gas per 24 hours with a mean of 600 ml. This averages out to 13.6+/−6 passages per 24 hours. The basal flatal rate (also referred to as the BFR in private circles) averages 15ml. per hour but substantially increases after one ingests a meal. For example, following a standard meal, one notes an increase in the flatal rate. This rate, medically speaking, is referred to as the PPFR, or Post-Prandial Flatal Rate, and averages approximately 100 ml per hour. Hence, riding in a crowded elevator immediately after dining is contraindicated. To add fuel to the fire, so to speak, how about a picnic with hot dogs and baked beans? Have you ever pondered over the rationale for eating hot dogs and beans OUTDOORS? Baked beans cause the PPFR to increase to 176ml/hour.

* * *

The release of methane into the earth's atmosphere contributes to a phenomenon called the greenhouse effect. This greenhouse effect, a gradual warming of the earth caused by excessive carbon dioxide, has long been attributed to the industrial revolution. However, another source of methane happens to be flatulent sheep, reports a geophysicist from the New Zealand Institute of Nuclear Sciences. This is obviously a significant problem in New Zealand, a country with a population of 70 million sheep. Those 70 million sheep release 2.5 billion gallons of methane into the earth's atmosphere every week. The same researcher noted that if you hooked up a sheep to the carburetor of a car, you could run it for several kilometers a day. To power the same vehicle by people, you need a whole football team and a couple of kegs of beer.

* * *

The September 1986 journal, *Surgery,* published a fascinating review article entitled, "Rectal foreign bodies: Case reports and a comprehensive literature review" that revealed that no less than 700 identified objects had been removed from approximately 200 rectums— a walloping 3.5 items per butt. Note that those are just the objects that have been identified. It doesn't mention those objects that couldn't be identified. One case was particularly interesting. A 38-year-old male reported an assault by a so-called friend, and after all was said and done, the following items were removed from the rectum: one pair of spectacles, a suitcase key, a tobacco pouch, and some reading material, a magazine (they didn't say which one). An interesting combination of items, wouldn't you agree?

Foods were found to be popular items for rectal consumption—the most common were:

Carrots and cucumbers (numbers 1 and 2 on the list)

Bananas, onions (Vidalia, I hope), and zucchini—all tied for the number 3 spot.

Other popular items were sticks or broom handles, as were bottles and jars. Actually, jars of perfume were found quite often.

Miscellaneous items included a cattle horn (mooo), a frozen pig's tail (you got me on that one), an ice pick (owww), tin cup (they didn't say if there was money in it), spatula, toothbrush holder, and baby powder can...just to name a few.

Some of the situations reported by the patients as to how the items arrived in the rectums were very original. One man inserted an entire jar of cold cream plus a lemon to relieve the itching of hemorrhoids. Interestingly enough, hemorrhoids were nowhere to be found when the cold cream jar and lemon were extracted. Perhaps this is a new cure for hemorrhoids, unbeknownst to the medical field.

One group of workers who are at high risk for the accidental insertion of objects in the rectum are in the agricultural field. Rectal impalement in this group is fairly common compared to lawyers and such, and the objects involved included pitchfork handles, hay hooks, stakes, shovel handles, fence pickets, animal horns, tree branches, iron bars, and chair legs. Need I say more?

* * *

Tobacco hasn't always been given such a bad rap as a cause of multi-system disease. In fact, in the early 1800s it was used therapeutically as a muscle relaxant. A strong cigar was introduced into the patient's rectum in order to relax the muscles prior to surgery. Some M.D.'s dispensed with the formality of placing a cigar in the rectum and would either blow smoke directly into the rectum or inject tobacco distillates into the blood. Hmmm—sort of gives a new meaning to the term smokin'.

* * *

Well, here's one of those time honored traditions that has not been questioned in 100 years—which end of the rectal suppository should be inserted first?

Traditional insertion technique recommends the apex (thick bulbous head), enter the rectum first. However, a study on 100 subjects (60 adults and 40 children) compared apical vs. base insertion and found that 59 adults and 39 children preferred base insertion over apical. Besides patient preference, two other advantages were found. One, there was no need to insert the finger into the rectal canal when the base was inserted first, and two, the incidence of expulsion (3 total) occurred with apical insertion. The authors of the study (*Lancet*, Vol. 338, 1991) suggest that the arrangement of the muscles around the anal canal and rectum facilitate the insertion of the torpedo-shaped suppository with the base first.

*   *   *

GREAT MOMENTS IN MEDICAL HISTORY
5

D octors are whippersnappers in ironed white coats
Who spy up your rectums and look down your throats.
And press you and poke you with sterilized tools,
And stab at solutions that pacify fools.
I used to revere them and do what they said
Till I learned what they learned on was already dead.

—Gilda Radnor
(*New England Journal of Medicine*, Nov. 17, 1988)

*   *   *

The feat of David felling the giant Goliath may be
attributed to endocrine pathology. The endocrine abnormalities

may have included functioning tumors of the parathyroid and pituitary glands. Evidence to support:

1   Functioning parathyroid tumors produce excessive amounts of parathyroid hormone (PTH). PTH mobilizes calcium from bone resulting in "brown" tumors, or softening of bones. How else could a measly stone from a homemade slingshot have penetrated the skull bone with such velocity as to cause sudden death?

2   A functioning tumor of the pituitary gland may produce excess amounts of growth hormone resulting in giantism. Pituitary tumors extending beyond the base of the brain turcica may also compress the optic chiasm. Compression of the optic chasm results in the loss of peripheral vision, not being able to see someone approaching from the side. As a result, Goliath would have had a partial loss of vision which may have contributed to his demise.

*   *   *

You all have undoubtedly heard of Dr. Charles-Edourd Brown-Sequard, a famous French physician practicing medicine in the mid-1800s. He is best known for his studies on a group of African tribal members who punished misconduct by taking a small, thin, sharp knife and hemi-secting the spinal cord of the perpetrator. Hence, the term Brown-Sequard syndrome, used to describe the signs and symptoms seen with hemi-section of the spinal cord.

A less known discovery by Dr. Brown-Sequard was one made in the spring of 1889. He was 72 at the time and feeling rather weak, old, and debilitated. He decided this feeling would never do, so he rejuvenated himself with a fluid extracted from the crushed testicles of a young canine friend. After 10 injections of his special potion, which he termed "testicular extract," he was feeling quite chipper again. He was racing up and down stairs, and he noted in his diary that he could "shoot a jet of urine a fourth again as far as he could before his injections." Quite an accomplishment wouldn't you say?

Within a year of Brown-Sequard's claims of increased energy and virility, physicians from Bangkok to Bangor, Maine were giving testicular extract for whatever ailed ya'. It was touted as the cure all for senile feebleness, cancer, seizures, leprosy, and cholera just to name a few.

Although many of his fellow colleagues failed to support his ideas and simply brushed them aside as delusions, others began to see the usefulness of glandular extracts in the treatment of deficiencies of the various glands.

Two years later an English M.D. treated a woman with end-stage thyroid disease with juice from a sheep's thyroid. She promptly recovered, thus confirming Brown-Sequard's theory that body organs secreting active substances could be used to treat certain deficiencies.

* * *

The metal, mercury, was once used in the silvering of mirrors and in the production of felt hats. The felt hat workers often developed toxic central nervous system changes, called madness; hence the phrase, "mad as a hatter," coined by Lewis Carroll in *Alice in Wonderland.*

* * *

The first cardiac catherizations were performed in 1929 by a German physician named Werner Forssman. He passed rubber tubes through the veins of the arm into the heart in cadavers, but decided to do the experiment on a live subject—himself. First attempts failed because the physician who had agreed to help him lost his nerve; the second attempt was with a nurse, probably Nurse Diesel, and it worked. With a fluoroscope and mirror, he followed the catheter's progress as he moved it up the vein of his own arm. When he had inserted the tube 20 inches (51 cm), its tip entered the right atrium. Since he knew that no one would believe him without absolute proof, he walked down the hall, climbed two flights of stairs, and had x-rays taken to prove his achievement. No mention was made as to whether or not he made it back down the two flights of steps, and back down the hall.

*　　*　　*　　*　　*

The curative powers of the common foxglove herb were first officially recognized in 1776. The principal of Brasenose College in Oxford, England was suffering from the classical entity known as "dropsy," a waterlogging of the tissues due to heart failure, more commonly referred to in this day and age as peripheral edema. He attempted all of the orthodox remedies prescribed by the physicians of that era, but nothing seemed to help. He finally abandoned the orthodox remedies and slugged down a special tea brewed by an elderly woman in the village of Shropshire. Lo and behold, he recovered with such amazing speed that the news spread throughout the land. A local M.D., William Withering, analyzed the herbal tea and found over 20 varieties of herbs; however, he also found that the active ingredient was foxglove, the Latin name of which is *digitalis*. Why digitalis? It has 5 leaves branching from the end of the stem that look like fingers, or digits.

*　　*　　*

Vincent Van Gogh may have suffered from pica, a craving for unusual substances or foods. Van Gogh's unnatural craving involved a liqueur called absinthe, which contains the chemical thujone, a substance distilled from plants such as wormwood. Thujone is toxic to the central nervous system. Not only did he crave the thujone-laced absinthe, but he was also known to crave substances such as camphor that contained chemicals known as terpenes which are also toxic to the central nervous system, and are known to trigger tonic-clonic seizures when ingested. Van Gogh had at least four documented tonic-clonic seizures the last eighteen months of his life. Letters from Van Gogh's colleagues substantiate his terpene fetish. One fellow artist had to restrain Van Gogh from swilling turpentine one evening. It was also a well-known fact that Van Gogh would nibble on his paints which also contained terpene.

* * *

Dietary treatment for pernicious anemia (a type of B_{12} deficiency) was first introduced in the early 1900s. Patients were required to consume at least a half a pound of liver per day as their treatment for this severe, unrelenting anemia. At the time (1926), this was heralded as a lifesaving miracle; however, the actual cause of the disease had not been elucidated. Approximately two years later, a research associate at Boston City Hospital named William Castle posed a very simple question, "Why don't normal people need one-half pound of liver per day to prevent the development of pernicious anemia?" Now William (who flunked his course in hematology while a med student at Harvard), knew that stomachs of patients with pernicious anemia were shriveled and atrophic, and he proposed that this may cause them to lack some very important factor that the stomach could no longer provide. How did he approach this question? His experimental protocol consisted of two consecutive periods of approximately 10 days, during which daily reticulocyte counts were made. (A rise in the reticulocyte count would indicate that new red blood cells were being produced in the bone marrow.) During the first period the patient received 200gm of rare hamburger steak daily (the rationale was that hamburger meat is similar to liver in texture). During this ten-day period there was no rise in the reticulocyte count.

During the second part of the protocol, Castle himself would consume 200 gm of hamburger meat and one hour later insert an NG tube to collect the partially digested contents and gastric juice. He would incubate these goodies for several hours until liquefaction of the meat occurred. He then inserted an NG tube in the patient and delivered the goodies to the patient. The patients showed a response: their reticulocyte counts began to rise, and their anemia responded as treatment continued.

Castle found that neither the hamburger nor the gastric contents, when given alone, would help the patient. They needed to be given the combination in order for the treatment to be effective. He referred to the hamburger meat as the extrinsic factor and the gastric contents as the intrinsic factor. And now you know the rest of the story—these are referred to today as B_{12} and intrinsic factor (also known as gastric binding protein).

P.S. You may be asking yourself, "Why did the one-half pound of liver work by itself, but not the hamburger by itself? Good question. Liver contains so much B_{12} that the mass effect of the shear amount of B_{12} given was enough to ensure sufficient absorption and clinical response despite the loss of the binding protein in the atrophic stomach.

* * *

Consider the career of the French phenomenon Joseph Pujol. Born in Marseille in 1857, his stage name was "Le

Petomane" (French, to break wind). Pujol mastered the sphincteric abilities of voluntary inspiration, retention, and voluntary exhalation, so to speak. To inhale, anal sphincter relaxation was combined with reduction of intra-abdominal pressure. The tighter the sphincter during exhalation, the higher the pitch and the lower the timbre.

He became known as the man with the musical anus, and his performances at the Moulin Rouge thrilled audiences between the years of 1892 and 1914. Bird trills, twitters, and warbles would precede an early version of what we know as "Name that Tune." Requests were honored for various passages and ditties of the day, including "au claire de la lune." The range of a Pujol symphony could extend from a brassy blare to a "violinistic tremolo." The grand finale was to blow out a candle from a one foot distance. His solo falsetto was such a hit that nurses had to revive the female portion of the audience. They passed out from laughing so hysterically that they developed "corset-induced" hysterical syncope.

*   *   *

In the late 1920s and early 1930s, veterinarians throughout the country warned farmers of "sweet clover disease." Cows that were eating spoiled and moldy sweet clover were dying from bleeding complications. In February, 1933, a Wisconsin dairy farmer packed up a bale of the spoiled, moldy sweet clover, a milk pail of blood, and his favorite deceased dairy cow, and drove to the University of Wisconsin to attempt to find the cause of the cow's death. After speaking with a University biochemist, Karl Link, he decided to leave the bale of clover for evaluation.

Six years and an infinite number of spoiled, moldy clover bales later, Link isolated the substance that made the cows bleed to death. He named it dicumarol, a derivative of a similar chemical known as coumarin, the substance that gives sweet clover its scent. Link also discovered its biochemical sequence and was able to reproduce it in the laboratory. The word spread like wildfire, and physicians all over the country were beating his door down to use it for their patients who had clotting problems. By 1944, dicumarol was used widely as an anti-clotting agent. One major problem, however, was that it was poorly absorbed from the GI tract, therefore blood levels were erratic and difficult to control.

Link continued to experiment with the substance by producing various strengths of dicumarol. He decided that one of the more potent strengths could be used as a rat poisoning agent. When the tasteless, odorless dicumarol was mixed with a grain, rats would devour it in large quantities, and would subsequently hemorrhage to death. This rodent killer was called "warfarin," and was available nationwide by 1951.

Shortly thereafter a young Army recruit decided that ingesting a box of warfarin would be a perfect way to commit suicide. He didn't die; however he did hemorrhage quickly—both internally and externally. His Army doctors concluded that the "rat warfarin" was absorbed much more rapidly than the "human dicumarol"—as evidenced by the patient's rapid hemorrhage. They began testing warfarin in humans—in small doses of course.

Four years later, President Dwight Eisenhower had a myocardial infarction while visiting Colorado. The Army physicians at Fitzsimmons Army Hospital in Denver decided to treat him with a "blood thinner", and they used small doses of rat poison rather than dicumarol, the approved drug for human consumption. Since the treatment was successful, warfarin became the oral anticoagulant of choice.

* * *

R$_X$UPDATE
6

H ow many times have you heard "I know it's gonna rain, I can feel it in my joints"? Naturally, the more you hear this, the more you wonder if there might be something to it. Research in the 1960s tested arthritis sufferers in a climate chamber and found that rising humidity and a falling barometric pressure—conditions associated with storms—did cause their joints to ache. Recent research confirmed the findings by having arthritis sufferers keep a diary of pain intensity for one year. They found that increasing humidity and decreasing barometric pressure also coincided with their pain patterns.

The cause of this phenomenon centers around the increased vascular permeability seen in arthritic patients. Since the intra-vascular pressure is higher than the pressure in the tissue wall, serum tends to be pushed into the tissues, and since the arthritic patient has a much "leakier" vascular wall than normal, serum tends to be pushed into the tissues of the joints. This movement of fluid from the vessels to the joint tissue would be greatest when the pressure of the surrounding environment is the lowest, as it is just before a storm. With the joints already stiff and swollen, the extra fluid may trigger the extra pain and stiffness.

*   *   *

A new topical preparation for the treatment of Herpes Zoster or shingles, as well as post-herpetic neuralgia has hit the market. The medicine is derived from capsium, the red peppers used to make chili pepper and cayenne pepper. Called capsaicin (Zostrix), the major side effect is burning of the skin where applied. That's nothing new for these patients—most of them have been complaining of burning in the area of the shingles prior to the treatment.

*   *   *

One 325mg tablet of Aspirin contains 70-90mg of sodium. This must be considered when administering to patients with essential hypertension or sodium retaining states such as congestive heart failure or renal failure.

*   *   *

Bloodletting for the purpose of treating disease caused by harmful "humors" has been utilized since before the days of Hippocrates. In the 1830s bloodletting reached its peak of popularity, and 20 million leeches a year were used as blood suckers.

*   *   *

A central venous catheter has become plugged. You don't have access to urokinase or streptokinase. What else might you try? How about 0.1 N Hydrochloric acid? Less than 1 ml of 0.1 N HCl acid will do the job especially if the plug is due to precipitation caused by drugs and calcium and phosphorus. It can also clear catheters occluded by thrombi. And, just in case you're worried about changing the serum pH—it would take 9 ml to change the bicarbonate level by 1mmol/L. Thus, the risk of inducing metabolic acidosis is negligible. (Shulman RJ: *J Parenteral Enteral Nutrit* 1988; 12:509).

* * *

A new study utilizing computerized pill bottles has confirmed how poorly Americans comply with taking their prescribed meds. The compliance rate was inversely proportional to the number of pills prescribed per day. For a once daily pill, the compliance rate was 81%. The compliance rate slipped from 81% to 77% with a three times a day regimen and fell dramatically to 39% with a four times a day regimen. Clearly, the data demonstrates how difficult a four times a day regimen is to maintain.

* * *

Prescription non-compliance leads to an estimated 125,000 deaths, 20 million lost work-days, and thousands of hospitalizations per year. One study showed that 93% of the patients who fill their initial prescriptions, only 68% return for the refill when ordered, and 15% stop taking their first prescription prematurely.

* * *

The National Cancer Institute's drug development program receives more than 20,000 compounds yearly. Of that number, 10,000 are selected for screening. The pre-screening process yields approximately 350 compounds of which 250 are suitable for testing in animal experiments. This process leads to about 20 "actives" of which 10 may proceed to production and development. Seven to nine will advance to toxicology studies, and only five to eight survive to qualify for clinical trials.

*   *   *

It seems as though every month we find a new use for the beta blocker Propanalol (also known as Inderal). Listen to this one...PROPANALOL CONTRACEPTIVE PILLS PER VAGINA! Yes, take 80mg every evening from the last day of your menstrual period until the first day of your next menstrual period without fail. It appears as if more drug is absorbed through the mucous membrane of the vagina than the GI tract, and both isomers of the drug are spermacidal. There is an extra added benefit. If you are hypertensive your blood pressure will also be reduced. Yes indeed, Propanalol per vagina also causes the systemic beta blocking effects that it does by mouth: reduced BP and reduced pulse rate. As a spermicide it appears to be as effective as foams, jellies, etc. There was a 4% failure rate with Propanolol as compared to a 3-5% failure rate for other spermicides; a 2% failure rate for diaphragm + spermicide; and a 2-20% failure rate for natural family planning.

*   *   *

A word of caution concerning the application of topical cortico-steroids (hydrocortisone)—the absorption varies with body location. If topical steroids are applied to the face and scalp there is a 5-10 times greater systemic delivery than if applied to the forearm. The genital skin, especially the scrotum, has up to 50 times more absorption than the forearm vs. the palms and soles of the feet with their thick stratum corneum. These areas have one-fifth the absorption of the forearm. Steroid penetration of the skin is enhanced 5-100 times if the skin is hydrated, so patients should be instructed to apply steroid cream after bathing when skin surfaces are still moist. Steroid penetration is also increased through inflamed skin. The third factor related to steroid absorption is the vehicle through which the steroid molecule is delivered. Ointments achieve better effects than creams or lotion preparations of the same steroids.

* * *

The temperatures inside a glove compartment can reach 50° higher than the outside temperature. If it's 85°F outside

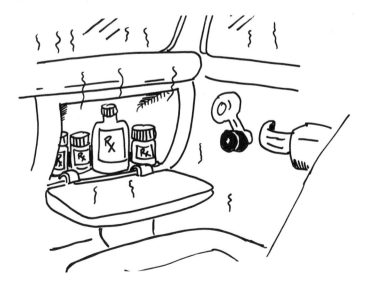

the glove compartment temperature is 110°F; if it's 100°F outside, the glove compartment temperature is 150°F.

Since storage temperature for medications should not exceed 86°F, the best place to keep meds in the car while you're running an errand, is on the floor. Floor temperature is 20 degrees cooler than the glove compartment, and it is even more effective if you throw some item (like a newspaper) over them.

* * *

Arsenic was probably the first substance banned as an occupational hazard. As long as 5,000 years ago, Bronze Age metal workers stopped smelting arsenic because of its adverse side effects which included pain, numbness, and weakness in the legs. This explains why the Greek, Roman, and Germanic gods of metalworking were all portrayed as lame.

Arsenic does not have a totally bad reputation. It was discovered to be effective against syphilis in 1909 by Dr. Paul Ehrlich.

* * *

The history of the evolution of nitroglycerin as the major component of dynamite to a major treatment for angina pectoris is an interesting one. Following World War II, large numbers of workers from munitions plants suddenly began dying from myocardial infarctions. Their deaths came shortly after the closure of the munitions plant as they were beginning careers in other areas. Apparently, many of these workers had been inhaling the nitrate compounds while they worked at the munitions plant making nitroglycerin for bombs. Their arteries were in a constant state of vasodilation therefore, the symptoms of coronary artery disease were masked. Soon after leaving the munitions plant for other jobs, their protection via nitrate fumes was gone, and their heart problems quickly surfaced.

By the way, dynamite is 75% nitroglycerin compared to less than 1% in a nitroglycerin tablet, just in case you were wondering why patients didn't blow up when they took their NTG tabs. (P.S., don't keep your nitroglycerin tablets in a hot glove compartment.)

And speaking of nitroglycerin, a gentleman from Georgia noted that the nitrate skin patches he wore on his chest to control angina (due to the nitrate's ability to vasodilate) gave him a pounding headache, but the patch, when worn on the leg, did not induce pounding headaches. He decided to experiment one day and rubbed a nitrate patch on his penis. Within 5 minutes, his penis had vasodilated, so to speak, inducing an erection, and he had sexual intercourse with his wife. Within minutes, the Ms. developed a pounding headache. She was not amused when he explained his experimentation with the patch.

Medical science has benefited from his experimentation. We now know that nitrates, when rubbed on strategic areas, can induce vasodilation to the advantage of the patient. We also know that the systemic effects can be absorbed through the vaginal mucosa in large enough amounts to induce cerebral vasodilation and cause a pounding headache.

*　　*　　*

Feverfew, an herbal remedy for migraine headaches, significantly reduces the frequency as well as the accompanying nausea and vomiting associated with the headache. In addition, it decreases the severity of the attacks, but does not alter the duration of the migraine. Although the mechanism of action is not well delineated, it is hypothesized that a specific substance in the plant (sesquiterpene lactone, for those of you who are trivia buffs) reduces the ability of platelets to release their vasoactive peptides. The release of vasoactive peptides such as serotonin from platelets is one of the postulated causes of migraine headaches. (*Lancet* 1988; Jul 23; 2:189-92.)

* * *

Recent studies have correlated the reduction of blood pressure with the watching of fish in an aquarium. Hypertensive, as well as non-hypertensive volunteers in a study published by the University of Pennsylvania watched fish in an aquarium for a specified length of time. The blood pressure of the non-hypertensive volunteers dropped as they observed the fish, and the blood pressure of the volunteers with hypertension dropped even more. This study did not go unobserved. Entrepreneurs in the video tape business quickly developed 30- minute tapes of tropical fish complete with the sound effects of a home aquarium. The benefits? Hypertensive patients don't have to worry about pushing their blood pressure back up by having to contend with all of the worry, mess, and bother of taking care of a home aquarium.

* * *

Spider angiomas appear to be secondary to estrogen excess in patients with liver disease. True spider angiomas have a central feeder vessel with surrounding "legs" radiating from the central feeder. The spider angioma will blanch with central pressure. The presence of five spider angiomas or less in a premenopausal female is a variation of normal, especially in the pregnant female. However, one lousy spider angioma in a male is considered abnormal. In patients with acute fulminant hepatitis secondary to viral infections, drug toxicity, or CCL_4 poisoning, large numbers of spider angiomas can appear over a short period of time. Spider angiomas are seen primarily above the nipples.

* * *

Oral temperatures taken with an electronic thermometer provide the best indicator of "core" temperature. Rectal temps are usually 0.3-0.6 degrees Centigrade (.05-1.0 degree Farenheit) higher than oral, and this has been attributed in part to heat generation by bacteria within the rectum and colon. Contrary to popular belief, rectal temps are no more accurate a reflection of core temperature than are properly measured oral temperatures. False oral readings can result from smoking, eating or drinking hot liquids, vigorous exercise, chewing, and mechanical manipulation of the mercury thermometer during measurement. In the true sense of the word, a "core temperature" would be taken from the right atrium or duodenum. So neither the oral nor rectal temperature is a core temperature, they are superficial temperatures.

* * *

The pulse rate during periods of hyperthermia can provide a reliable indication of the physiologic importance of fever.

The heart rate normally increases 10-20 beats per minute for every 0.6 degrees Centigrade (1.0 degrees Farenheit) higher rise in temperature. Absence of such an increase, along with a rapid decrease in fever without accompanying sweating, suggests factitious fever. However, certain conditions may be present with bradycardia and fever and should be sought in patients with FUO (fever of unknown origin). Some examples include Legionnaire's Disease, myceplasma infection, mumps, psittacosis, Salmonella typhi infection, infectious hepatitis, heart disease, and increased intracranial pressure. In addition, Beta blockers such as Inderal can keep the pulse low when a patent has a temperature.

* * *

The neurotransmitter in the hypothalamus that regulates fever is dopamine. Increased levels of dopamine increase the temperature setting mechanism and fever is the end result. Thorazine blocks dopamine receptors in the hypothalamus and will decrease the temperature. Schizophrenic patients receiving dopamine tend to have lower body temperatures for this reason.

* * *

Bacteria are now used in the manufacture of antibiotics, vitamins, vaccines, and hormones, and are involved at some point in the production of 20% of all prescription drugs.

* * *

The classic picture of atropine poisoning: "Hot as a hare, blind as a bat, dry as a bone, red as a beet, and mad as a hatter."

We may be applying special eye drops to the eyes in the near future. The special drops being tested are the equivalent of sunglasses or sun block to protect the cornea. The drops block out 98% of the ultraviolet light for 3-4 hours and should be available within the year.

* * *

A new female urinal called the "She-inal" is a hand-held funnel that fits snugly over the area involved. A dispenser provides a biodegradable paper cover for each user. It takes up ½ the space of a regular toilet, the user can stand without having to undress so much (clothes can be pulled to the side) and last but not least—this may be the solution to the long lines to the ladies room.

* * *

MEDICAL MORSELS
7

W
hen do phobias rear their ugly heads? Recent research shows that it actually depends on the phobia. On the average, the fear of animals (zoophobia) begins at age 7, the fear of blood at age 9, the fear of dentists at age 12, the fear of close spaces (claustrophobia) at age 20, and fear of open spaces (agoraphobia) at age 28.

*   *   *

Why are pygmys pygmys? Why are they smaller than other people from birth to death? At age 10 they virtually stop growing and they have no growth spurt at puberty as does the rest of the population. The failure to grow is due to a lack of the hormone IGFI, an insulin-like growth factor. (*New England Journal of Medicine*; 9/10/87.)

*   *   *

If the cerebral cortex were flattened out it would cover over two square feet.

*   *   *

The world's oldest living man lived to the ripe old age of 120 years and 237 days. He decided to stop smoking 2 years after his first heart attack, at age 114.

*   *   *

Those little flecks and threads you see floating around in your eyes actually have a fancy Latin name: *muscae volitantes*, meaning "fluttering flies." Almost everyone experiences these so called floaters; however, the phenomenon is most common in near-sighted individuals. The threads are believed to be the remnants of the embryologic hyloid artery that nourished the lens and eye during fetal development. The artery disintegrates prior to birth, but some of the remnants may remain forever floating in the vitreous humor. Floaters are usually benign and tend to increase as we age.

*   *   *

In the growth phase, scalp hairs lengthen a third of a millimeter per day on average, or 5 inches per year. Hair grows fastest between the ages of 15 and 30, and women's hair grows faster than men's. Hair also grows faster in the summer, in tropical climates, and when the skin is irritated. This is probably due to an increased blood supply to the scalp skin under all of these conditions. Prolonged irritation of the skin also seems to increase growth, again because of increased blood to the area.

This may explain the bushier, thicker hair on arms and legs that have been in casts, the newly shaved armpit, or facial hair that goes through a growth spurt, and the patches of longer, thicker hair on the shoulders of workers carrying heavy packs with straps. Uncut over a lifetime, a head of hair could theoretically reach a length of 30 feet; however, the current record is 26 feet, set in 1949 by none other than Swami Pandarasannadhi of India.

* * *

As a matter of biology rather than sexism, if something bites you, it is probably female.

* * *

In 1985 the American population globbed 1,300,000 gallons of suntan lotion on their exposed epidermis.

* * *

One of the great barroom legends popularized by the movie, *You Only Live Twice,* was that Sumo wrestlers have the ability to "will" their testicles to ascend into their abdomen (inguinal canal). This is probably not true, although this is not physiologically impossible. Moles, hedgehogs, and shrews do it on a daily basis; however, no one is quite sure why. Back to the original story. In humans, the testes are suspended from the cremasteric muscle, which is controlled by the autonomic (involuntary) nervous system. This muscle raises and lowers the testicles as necessary to keep the temperature-sensitive sperm at a constant simmer. Under certain stimuli, such as a cold shower, or more entertainingly, a gentle stroking on the inside of the upper thigh, the "cremasteric reflex" takes over and the testes are partially retracted into the body.

It's been shown that automatic functions such as blood pressure and pupillary constriction can be consciously controlled through yoga and the like, and presumably the same could be done with the testicles.

* * *

Here are a few interesting laws still on the books in various cities throughout the U.S.:
- Bluff, Utah: The law forbids barbers from eating onions between 7 a.m. and 7 p.m.

- Wakefield, R.I.: Citizens are banned from entering a movie theater within four hours after eating garlic.
- Sutherland, Iowa: Citizens may not carry ice-cream cones in their pockets.
- Halstead, Kansas: Residents must refrain from eating ice cream with a fork in public.
- Redbush, Kentucky: It is against the law for any citizen to be seen riding an ugly horse.

* * *

Every minute of the day a teenager gets a sexually transmitted disease.

* * *

The bad news: each minute of our lives 300 million cells die. The good news: we replace lost cells as fast as they die. The final news: if we didn't replace the cells we would be dead in 230 days.

* * *

The everyday sit-up burdens the lumbar vertebrae with as much pressure as deep-sea divers feel at 570 feet. A high jump may load the femur with approximately 20,000 pounds of stress upon landing. The bones of the feet must suffer the body's weight during each of the 19,000 steps an average person takes each day.

* * *

A tourist recently set off the security system at the White House. Shortly before entering he had taken an exercise stress test in which the radioisotope, thallium was administered.

* * *

A new five minute laser procedure produces scarring and stiffening of the back of the soft palate. This keeps it from vibrating and puts an end to snoring in even the worst cases.

The procedure has been successfully performed on 20 patients in Great Britain.

* * *

The average child watches between 23 and 27 hours of TV per week and sees an estimated 1,000 murders, 20,000 commercials, and 15,000 sexual encounters.

* * *

Compression of the breasts for mammography requires 25-40 pounds of pressure.

* * *

Only 4% of U.S. adults believe they have gum disease, whereas 75% actually do.

* * *

Older mothers have a higher probability of having children who are lefties, according to a group of researchers from the University of British Columbia in Vancouver. Mothers who are 40 and over are twice as likely to have left-handed children. The researchers speculate that older mothers have more stressful pregnancies and deliveries, and that prenatal stress contributes to left-handedness.

* * *

Cleveland Clinic researchers have found a woman with uncombable hair syndrome, a disorder in which head hair grows so unruly it can't be managed by normal means. Not even conditioners or industrial strength mousse can control this monster. It appears as if a cross-section of a strand of this hair is triangular or bean-shaped instead of round, and stands straight out like it hasn't been brushed for years.

* * *

Virginia state records list the following surnames given to children: Salts, Alien, Navel, New Fang, Nicey Horsie, Molegold, Comfort Care, Turnip Seed and Cigarette.

* * *

Eighty percent of mothers cradle their infants in their left arm. Regardless of culture or where she lives, this seems to be a universal trait. In fact, gorillas and chimpanzees frequently cradle their infants and more than 80% of the time they do it on the left side. Many theories have been proposed as to why this left-handed preference occurs. One proposed that it leaves Mom's right hand free for opening doors and baby jars, which sounds feasible, until studies revealed that left-handed women also show the same left-cradling preference. The second theory suggests that babies held on the left are soothed by the maternal heartbeat; however, the sound is mostly inaudible in this position. The third theory has been recently proposed by two researchers from the University of Liverpool. Their findings suggest that the left-cradling dates back 6-8 million years. Such long endurance of the habit would suggest that it provides a survival advantage. They speculate that emotion-laden information is handled by the brain's right side. The right side of the brain has input from the left eye and ear, so that a mother holding her infant on the left side monitors the infant with her left eye and ear, while using her emotionally-savvy right brain. The research also suggests that left-arm cradling and right-brain baby-watching results in better bonding between mother and infant. This all results in a better chance of survival for the offspring.

* * *

On a more serious note, only 38% of the American population cleans their belly-button every day. Only?!

* * *

MEDICAL MINUTIAE

Half of the number of surgical sponges left in patients remain undiscovered for a period of five or more years after surgery.

*   *   *

Sexual intercourse occurs 100 million times daily around the world. This results in 910,000 conceptions and 350,000 cases of sexually transmitted disease per day. (WHO, June 1993.)

*   *   *

Japan will soon be installing high tech toilets built with biosensors that detect the amount of glucose in the urine.

*   *   *

Speaking of high tech from Japan—a Japanese company has developed a "singing condom" which plays the Beatles song, *Love Me Do,* at the appropriate moment. The base of the condom contains a microchip and works similar to the way a musical greeting card does—when you open it, it plays (no pun intended).

*   *   *

Women who pig out on a dinner date will probably NOT be asked out for dinner again. Researchers have found that women who eat like birds are perceived (by both men and women) as more feminine and better looking than those who eat heartily. Of course, a measure of masculinity is how well they can "pack it away."

*   *   *

The American Automobile Association reports that by the time a child is 16, he/she has seen approximately 100,000 beer commercials.

*   *   *

Driving under the influence (DUI) of alcohol carries numerous penalties in our country including monetary fines, probation and the suspension of one's driver's license. All seem to be horrible and severe punishments to those being punished. However, they don't know how easily they're being let off. A DUI in the Soviet Union will result in a lifetime suspension of the driver's license. In El Salvador or Bulgaria citizens never need to worry about a DUI again, because they'll be executed by a firing squad after the first DUI. Sweden and Finland commit you to one year in jail at hard labor. Norway only gives you three weeks of hard labor and a one-year driver's license suspension. In South Africa you might as well pack your duffel bag—you're going to jail for 10 years, or you'll get a $10,000 fine, or you might even get both.

* * *

People who drink three to four alcoholic drinks per day should never take more than two grams of Tylenol per 24-hour period. Alcohol induces Tylenol to be degraded by the liver into metabolic by-products that are hepatotoxic. As a result, both drugs are synergistic in their harmful effects on the liver.

* * *

The philtrum is that little depression between the two ridges under the nose. Can you believe it has a name? Almost every animal has a philtrum—even lizards. The ridges are actually there for a reason; they protect a particularly sensitive spot in the skull where three bones meet: two from the sides and one from the top. (The one from the top is the one that keeps your nostrils separate.) If the ridges fail to develop in the human, you have a child born with a cleft lip.

Another fact about the philtrum. The word is derived from the Greek *philtron,* meaning "love charm." The ancient Greeks thought that the lips resembled the shape of Cupid's bow, the

MEDICAL MINUTIAE

philtrum then, metaphorically represented the grip, the center of Cupid's power.

* * *

Definitions:
- **The perfect stool**—twice around the pan and pointed at both ends.
- **The ultimate Generalist**—He learns less and less about more and more until he can tell you almost nothing about everything.

* * *

Medical Meanings:
- **Hymen**—From the Greek *hymen,* a skin or membrane. The Greek word was used for all sorts of membranes, including the pericardium and peritoneum. Later Hymen became the name of the God of Marriage, a sort of overgrown Cupid. It was not until the 16th century that "hymen" was restricted to denote the vaginal or virginal membrane.
- **Hiccup**—An imitative word that when pronounced, sounds like what it means. Similar sounding words of the same meaning occur in most European languages. For Example: Spanish-hipo; French-hoquet; German-schluken. However the medically correct term is the rather stuffy word "singultus."
- **Hysterectomy**—Derived from the combination of the Greek *hystera,* the womb or uterus, and *tome,* a cutting. To the Greeks, *hysterikos* meant a suffering in the womb. As far back as Plato's era the uterus was described as becoming "indignant, dissatisfied, and ill-tempered and it caused a general disturbance of the body until it became pregnant." This teaching gave rise to the age-old tendency to attribute various abnormal

manifestations to specific body organs. Emotional instability, thought to be more characteristic of females was blamed on the uterus. From this anatomic designation comes the term hysteria and hysterical.

♦ **Nostril**—This term is related to the common word "thrill." The Middle English *thrillen* originally meant to pierce. Nostril use to be spelled "nosethrill," a hole pierced in the nose.

* * *

Do you ever just pick up "one last item" at the grocery store while waiting in line at the check-out counter? You're not the only one—the weekly sales per square foot near the cash registers in the average supermarket is $22.80 whereas the weekly sales per square foot elsewhere in the store is $7.76.

* * *

Vampires and werewolves may have a physiological basis. A Canadian chemist has correlated the appearance and actions of vampires and werewolves with an extreme form of the disease known as porphyria, an inherited red blood cell metabolic disorder. Individuals with porphyria appear to have paws instead of hands. Their lips and gums are so taut that their teeth become very prominent. Their skin is hypersensitive to sunlight (hence, they abhor the sun as vampires of lore traditionally did). A treatment for the disease is a red blood cell pigment known as heme. However, since blood infusions were not available in the Middle Ages, the next best thing was to drink a lot of blood and the neck of an unsuspecting victim seemed to be the best place to start. Victims suffering from porphyria also react adversely to a chemical in garlic, reputed in folklore to ward off werewolves and vampires.

* * *

The largest tumor ever recorded was an ovarian cyst removed from a woman in Texas. It weighed 328 pounds.

* * *

The champion blood donor in the world is none other than Allen Doster. He donated 1,800 pints or 225 gallons over a 20-year period between 1966 and 1986.

*   *   *

The longest beard ever grown by a woman was 14 inches. Good ole' Janice Deveree of Bracken County Kentucky.

*   *   *

Binney and Smith, the folks who make crayons, turn out more than two billion every year. If you were to lay all of those crayons end to end, they would circle the earth's equator four times. That distinctive, familiar crayon smell is produced by stearic acid, a saturated fat that comes from beef fat. Recently stearic acid has been shown to actually reduce cholesterol levels. Do you think one day we'll be taking not only an aspirin a day, but perhaps following it up with your choice of crayon?

And one more fascinating fact for you crayon fanatics—Binney and Smith no longer produce the color "FLESH" (which back in the early days was a pinkish color that we used on everyone's skin, the assumption being that everyone was pink). Since it is obvious that this is not true, the color "FLESH" has been deleted from all boxes of crayons. (I bet those flesh crayons will be collector's items one day.)

*   *   *

Moonshine is being produced in old car radiators these days, and these radiators have been soldered with lead. Folks who have been imbibing in moonshine from these old radiators have had lead levels as high as 259 micrograms/dl (levels higher than 156 micrograms/dl must be reported to state authorities for monitoring). Irreversible renal and neurologic damage can occur at 30-40 micrograms/dl and levels greater than 200 are rarely reported even in the most serious cases of occupational lead poisoning. Chelation therapy was needed in three of nine patients admitted to the hospital after imbibing in radiator-distilled moonshine.

*   *   *

Over a lifetime, the average American spends one year looking for misplaced objects.

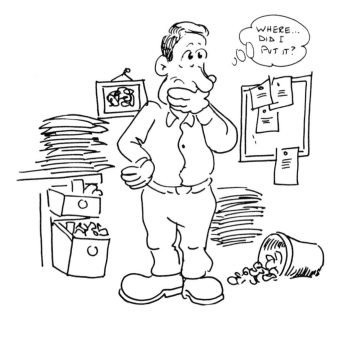

*   *   *

Eighteen MILLION Americans consume twenty-one TONS of aspirin each day.

*   *   *

An incredible statistic has emerged: a walloping 8,176 toothpick-related injuries occurred annually between the years of 1979-1982, or an annual rate of 3.6 per 100,000.

*   *   *

Many cultures originally used cultivated grains to measure short distances—in particular, the barleycorn had seeds of surprisingly consistent length. Three barleycorns placed end-to-end equaled exactly one inch. This led to the landmark decision by King Edward II of England. He decreed in 1324 that 36 barleycorns would equal one foot, and the rest is history.

* * *

A one-half pack per day smoker takes 35,000 puffs per year.

* * *

The Casket, a journal published in 1833, reported that snorting powdered moss scraped from decaying skulls would dispel headaches.

* * *

We have at any given time, 25 trillion red blood cells, 35 billion white blood cells, and 1.5 trillion platelets circulating through our blood vessels.

* * *

Do not mix household cleaning products. A 72-year-old woman in Oregon died from chlorine gas poisoning while scrubbing her bathtub. She had mixed a combination of bleach, cleanser, ammonia, and drain cleaner.

* * *

Glenn Warden, chief surgeon at Cincinnati's Shriners Burns Institute, has been cleared in an ethics panel probe after he drew smiling faces on the genital areas of two patients. The hospital wouldn't comment on the probe, however Warden stated that he drew "happy faces" on a 22 year-old man's genitals and on a woman's lower abdomen with their consent in order to relieve their tension about surgery.

* * *

With the average price of cigarettes at $2.00, the two-pack-a-day smoker spends $1,460 a year on cigarettes. In 20 years, the same smoker would have shelled out $29,000 on cigarettes alone—and in 30 years, $43,800.

*   *   *

One cannot catch a cold at the North Pole in the winter. Neither can one contract the flu, nor most of the diseases transmitted by viruses and germs. The winter temperature is so low in this part of the world that none of the standard disease-causing organisms can survive.

*   *   *

Henry Ward Beecher, when asked on his deathbed if he could raise his arm, answered "Well, high enough to hit you, Doctor."

*   *   *

From the *Arkansas Medical Dictionary*:
    Artery—the study of paintings
    Barium—what you do when patients die
    Bowel—a letter like a, e, i, o, u
    Cauterize—had eye contact with her
    D&C—where Washington is
    Enema—not a friend
    Node—was aware of
    Urine—opposite of "you're out"

*   *   *

Research psychologists from the University of Oklahoma have completed their perusal of 4,306 questionnaires filled out by high school youths. Their findings: Most youths (male, female, white, black) seem to have lost their virginity in the summer. June to be exact.

Possible reasons? The Raging Summer Hormones Theory: hormones rage more freely when it's hot outside and when the days are long. Or, The Summer Vacation Theory: school is out, jobs are scarce, hangin' out is in, and opportunities abound in the back seat and under the bushes.

*   *   *

The average number of times Americans touch one another while talking for one hour in a coffee shop is two. Puerto Rican friends touch each other an average of 180 times during that same hour. English friends don't touch at all, and the French touch 110 times.

*   *   *

Being involved in sports may be an extremely effective form of birth control. High school girls who are involved in sports are 80% less likely to become pregnant than girls who aren't involved in sports. Another added benefit—girls involved in sports are three times more likely to get their high school diploma than non-participants.

*   *   *

To protect yourself from magnetic fields you should stay 5 feet away from your microwave, 1½ feet away from a high intensity lamp, 16 inches from an electric clock, 3 feet from a hair dryer, and 12 inches from an electric shaver. Oh yes, and also 3 feet from an electric blanket. Three feet from a hair dryer? It would take you three hours to dry your hair. Twelve inches from and electric shaver?

*   *   *

The least healthy states in the nation are Alabama, Arkansas, Kentucky, Mississippi, Nevada, Pennsylvania, and West Virginia. The District of Columbia is also on the list. The ranking, made by the American Public Health Association, was based on five main categories—access to medical care, healthy environments, healthy neighborhoods, health behaviors, and community health services. The healthiest states are Hawaii, Maryland, New York, Vermont, Virginia, and Washington.

*　*　*

Given a choice of being obese again or having a leg amputated, 91% of 47 formerly obese men and women preferred amputation and 89% would prefer being blind. One hundred percent said they would rather be dyslexic, deaf, diabetic, or have heart disease than be obese.

*　*　*

SEX & CONTRACEPTION
8

C amels have the distinction of being the first animals to use IUDs. For years camel drivers placed apricot pits in the uteri of the females so that they would not become pregnant on long caravan trips.

What is the best form of contraception for humans? (Obviously the apricot pit will not do.) In order of failure rate, i.e. the number of pregnancies per 100 woman years:
1   abstinence (0)
2   sterilization of the male or female (.001)
3   birth control pills (.3)
4   diaphragm (1.9)
5   condom (3.60)
6   withdrawal (6.7)
7   spermacides (11.9)
8   rhythm method (15.5)

Condoms not only help to prevent pregnancy, they also help to prevent sexually transmitted diseases. Since 1987, the U.S. FDA has allowed condom manufacturers to list a roster of diseases that condoms, when properly utilized, can help prevent: gonorrhea, syphilis, chlamydia, herpes, and AIDS. However, be advised that 5% of all condoms sold in the U.S. are so-called "skin condoms," made from the cecum of a lamb. (Isn't it nice that we find uses for the most obscure animal parts?)

Anyway, these expensive "skin condoms" have been thought to produce a more "natural feel" than the traditional latex condom, and are the only form available for those allergic to latex. Unfortunately they contain large pores (up to 1.5 microns in size). This is smaller than a sperm, the size of Hepatitis B and larger than the AIDs virus. Thus, "Fourex Natural Skins" and "Trojan Kling-Tite Natural Lambs" may be fairly good contraceptives, but they are risky for the prevention of AIDS and hepatitis B transmission.

* * *

Here's an interesting study. Did you know that a woman who has only a daughter is 9% more likely to be separated or divorced than a woman with only a son. In two-child families, marriages were most stable when both children were boys. The risk of a broken family rose 9% when one of the two children was a girl, and 18% when both were girls. Why, one asks? University of Pennsylvania researchers found that fathers spend more leisure time with their sons than daughters and are more involved in making the rules for sons. The researchers hypothesize that because of the way men and women are socialized, there are more things for a father to do with a son. Therefore, fathers are drawn more closely into the family unit by a son.

* * *

A study of 62 U.S. Air Force "top gun" pilots who flew extended hours at high G forces fathered an abnormal 60:40 ratio of girls to boys. Two-hundred other officers not exposed to G forces had the normal 50:50 ratio. The relationship between high G force exposure and male fertility is being investigated.

* * *

Two types of allergic responses can occur during or after sexual intercourse. These reactions are due to an allergy to seminal fluid and include a localized reaction of burning pain, redness, and swelling of genital tissues, and a life-threatening systemic anaphylactic reaction with generalized itching, breathing difficulty, low blood pressure and shock. Localized reactions last from 24 to 48 hours and are most likely medicated by IgE anti-spermatozoal antibodies. This one deserves a comment. Let's say that your response to sexual intercourse was of the anaphylactic variety. Could you imagine the impending sense of doom that you feel whenever you see that little gleam in your partner's eyes? Do you load up on epinephrine and keep an O_2 tank at the bedside at all times? Are you having respiratory difficulty due to the pleasure you are receiving from the encounter, or are you gasping for breath due to widespread bronchoconstriction and lack of oxygen? Fortunately there is an answer to this complication. The use of condoms can prevent both the localized and the systemic responses by preventing contact between the vaginal mucosa and seminal fluid. However, if you want to become pregnant, epinephrine and O_2 at the bedside is the logical choice.

* * *

A recent study indicates that women kill their husbands for different reasons than men kill their wives. Of the women studied, all of them acted to stop a perceived imminent physical threat by husbands who repeatedly abused them. On the other hand, men who killed their wives had reacted violently to relieve stress resulting from their wives' threatened or actual withdrawal of emotional support.

* * *

The percentage of women between 20 and 40 who were infertile in 1965 was 4%; today that number is 11%. No one is quite sure why the number is increasing.

* * *

Ancient Egyptians realized that by blocking the passage of seminal fluid from entering the womb, a woman would not become pregnant. So they constructed their own diaphragm which consisted of a lint pad soaked in a mixture of acacia tips and honey. This mixture produces a profound amount of lactic acid, the active ingredient in most contraceptive jellies.

* * *

Contraception wasn't as popular in ancient Greece, however, the population was kept in check with the popular method of infanticide.

* * *

Who first invented the condom? You guessed it, the 16th century anatomist, Gabriel Fallopius (also responsible for naming the Fallopian tubes in the female). He actually designed a linen cap impregnated with oil to fit over the penis in order to help protect himself against the great pox—syphilis. Guess what Gabriel Fallopius died of.

Speaking of condoms, a report from the Trojan prophylactic factory states that condoms come in 2 sizes—7.1 inches by 52mm for the American market and 6.3 inches by 49mm for the Japanese market.

Condoms will deteriorate rapidly when exposed to ozone. Scanning electron micrographs of ozone-exposed condoms showed that their surface was covered with large craters and holes. The longer condoms are stored, the more damage from smog or ozone.

The percentage of condoms bought by females in 1975 was 15%, in 1986 that percentage rose to 40%. By the way, approximately 1 in 140 condoms will break when in use.

* * *

In an average day the prostate gland produces approximately one-tenth to four-tenths of a teaspoon of prostatic fluid. This is ordinarily drained into the urethra and excreted with urine. During periods of sexual arousal, the prostate pumps out about 3-10 times as much fluid as usual. If the man fails to have an orgasm, prostate fluid can back up in the prostate and cause congestion. This in turn can cause pain in the pelvic area along with painful and swollen testicles. The lay term for this condition is "blue balls"

* * *

The majority of the enzyme, acid phosphatase is found in the prostate gland and semen with only trace amounts in the liver, spleen, red blood cells, bone marrow, and platelets. Therefore, this enzyme is released into the serum with prostate damage and is present in ejaculated seminal fluid. The fact that acid phosphatase is found in the ejaculate can be an important clue in suspected sexual abuse cases. Finding acid phosphatase in vaginal secretions is a positive indicator of sexual intercourse. Greater than 50u per sample is considered semen positive. Acid phosphatase remains fairly constant in the vagina for approximately 14 hours after intercourse. Forty percent of percent of the women will be acid phosphatase positive after 24 hours and 11% will be positive after 72 hours. *Acid phosphatase* will be detected when spermatozoa are absent—such as after a vasectomy.

*   *   *

Halitosis (bad breath) can actually be due to cyclical changes induced by hormone fluctuations. Not only are you miserable with uterine cramping and the nagging problem of changing tampons and pads, but you can now add bad breath to the miseries of the monthly menses.

Bad breath rears its ugly head twice during your cycle; once during ovulation and again during menstruation. Around ovulation, a rise in estrogen trigger's shedding of the body's soft tissues, including those of the mouth. This increases the amount of debris that bacteria in the mouth can feast on. The more they feast, the worse your breath. Bacteria or oral flora, break down food particles and shed cells down into certain sulfur containing compounds that cause your *fetor oris* (Latin for fetid mouth.)

The longer the debris sits in the mouth, the longer the bacteria have to work, and the stronger the odor. (Smell your dental floss one day if you don't believe me—especially if you haven't flossed lately.) This is the reason why your breath doesn't smell like a bed of roses in the a.m. Bacteria do most of their work at night and you're not chewing or talking or allowing saliva to wash over the teeth and rid the mouth of debris.

*   *   *

In the U.S., Orientals have the highest rate of fraternal twins with one in 40 births; Caucasians have the lowest with one in 100; and African Americans fall in between with one in 77. The highest fraternal twinning rate is in Nigeria—one set of twins in every 20 births.

And speaking of twins, more women are having twins these days due to the fact that they are having babies later in life. In 1986, 21.6 of every 1000 babies were twins, as compared to 1980, when only 19.3 of every 1000 babies were twins. Why, you ask? Older women release more than one egg each month, as do women who use fertility drugs. Another reason for twins is the increased use of *in vitro* (test tube) fertilization.

*   *   *

Prior to 1900 most non-Jewish males were uncircumcised. The shift toward circumcision in this country was most likely the result of the Victorian obsession with masturbation, reinforced by the 1891 article by the British surgeon James Hutchinson, called "Circumcision as preventative of masturbation."

*   *   *

There are now do-it-yourself artificial insemination kits—featuring your basic turkey/meat baster as the major mode of sperm transportation.

*   *   *

The gender of a crocodile is determined purely by the weather. If it's hot outside it's a boy, if it's cold, well, it's a baby girl crocodile.

*   *   *

Estimated hours of work that are lost each year because of menstrual cramps: 576,000,000.

*   *   *

How often is an egg a lemon? It has been estimated that up to 60% of human pregnancies end in fetal wastage, and most wastage is believed to occur 4-5 weeks between conception and clinically recognized pregnancy. The causes of this fetal loss have recently been examined by Swedish obstetricians and geneticists. They studied women between the ages of 25 and 38 who were undergoing laparoscopy as a part of an infertility work-up. During this procedure the researchers aspirated ovarian follicles for examination under the light microscope. Their research found that nearly half of all oocytes collected from their sample of women had abnormal karyotypes. These chromosomally abnormal oocytes may well be responsible for the large number of spontaneous abortions and fetal wastage demonstrated. These may also account for the relatively low success rates achieved by programs of *in vitro* fertilization and embryo replacement. Corresponding studies on spermatozoa have demonstrated abnormal karyotypes in only 10%.

* * *

The female sea horse impregnates the male sea horse with about 600 eggs—he then washes his sperm over the eggs and fertilizes the group. About 50 days later the male sea horse begins labor and gives birth.

* * *

The only non-primates known to naturally menstruate are the elephant shrew and one species of bat—the *Glossaphage sorcinia*, just in case you're interested. And speaking of bats, (we'll get back to the menstruating elephant shrew later), Bracken Cave between San Antonio and Austin, Texas is said to contain an estimated 20 million bats—hopefully not the same species that menstruates.

* * *

The average woman loses about 2 ounces of blood and 17 mg of iron during her "monthly."

* * *

There are two types of impotence, one is physiologic and one is psychogenic. What is a simple, cheap, and effective way of differentiating between the two? The procedure is based on the concept of nocturnal tumescence, i.e., erections during sleep. Nocturnal erections are common and can only occur if all physiologic parameters are intact (that is, if everything is working properly). If an individual can experience an erection during the night, his impotence is most probably psychologic in origin. In other words, the nerves and blood supply are intact, and there is no known cause for the impotence. So, how can one determine psychologic vs. physiologic impotence without staying up all night and staring at "it"? Simple. Trek over to your friendly Post Office and buy 6 attached 1¢ stamps off the roll. Prior to bedtime, wet the stamps and wrap them around the base of the penis. Now, go to sleep, and when you wake, check the stamps. If they are separated, a nocturnal erection has occurred, and the problem is most likely psychogenic in origin.

* * *

The average length of sexual intercourse for humans is two, yes, I said two minutes. That doesn't seem like very long, but you can thank your lucky stars that you aren't a chimpanzee. The average length of intercourse for a couple of consenting chimpanzee adults is 7 seconds, yes, I said SECONDS.

* * *

A baby born in Ann Arbor, Michigan in 1986 was the first U.S. baby to be fathered via the process of electroejaculation. This method of conception is especially beneficial for men with spinal cord injury which renders them physiologically impotent.

(*Journal of the American Medical Association* 8/14/87:743-744)

* * *

A 1920's condom vending machine bears this message: "Should the presence of this machine be offensive to you, visit our hospitals, health institutes and asylums. You will be astounded. You may well place the blame upon yourself and others who think as you do."

* * *

In ancient times it was believed that evil spirits hovered over nurseries and that these evil spirits could be dispelled by certain colors that were presumed to combat evil. Blue was considered the most powerful color because of its association with the sky and heavenly spirits. Boys, in ancient times, were considered the most valuable child and blue clothing was considered as valuable, therefore girls were not swathed in blue clothing. Centuries later girls came into a color of their own, pink. Of course, this association stems from an old European legend which claims that baby girls were born inside pink roses.

* * *

If you kiss your beloved 3 times a day for one year you could potentially lose 2.8 pounds.

* * *

How can you tell that a girl is still a virgin? Here's a test devised by a Rabbi and recorded in the Talmud. His test consisted of seating two women, a virgin and a non-virgin, in turn, on a barrel of wine. The breath of the non-virgin smelled of wine, the breath of the virgin did not. It was presumed that the intact hymen prevented the odor of the wine ascending through the body. The idea obviously wasn't a sound anatomical one—the hymen blocks the reproductive tract, not the GI tract.

* * *

An interesting test for pregnancy in ancient Rome involved the measurement of the neck size of the woman presumed to be in "the family way." Thyroid enlargement occurs in pregnant women due to the increase in metabolism required to maintain the pregnancy and maintain energy throughout the pregnancy. The ancient physicians of Rome used to measure the neck daily in suspected pregnancies. The same procedure occurs in recorded medical literature of the 1700s in our country. A girl is a virgin when a string, which has been stretched from the tip of her nose to the end of her sagittal suture at the point where it joins the lambdoidal suture, can then wrap around her neck. If the string cannot reach all the way around, her thyroid is enlarged and she's in "the family way." And just think of all that money spent today on blood tests, ultrasounds, urine kits, etc., when a simple ball of string will do.

*   *   *

Various theories have been proposed as to the function of pubic and axillary hair. One such theory states that pubic and axillary hair gives something for babies to hold on to. Perhaps a more plausible explanation is that the hair helps to retain glandular secretions that are presumed to be powerful aphrodisiacs. Since when has the whiff of an armpit made you quiver with overwhelming desire?

Speaking of armpits, wait 'til you hear this one. Researchers at the University of Pennsylvania Chemical Senses Center have concluded from an amazing series of studies that male body odor plays a significant role in maintaining the health of the female reproductive system. How did they reach this interesting conclusion? The researchers collected underarm secretions from seven men and mixed this "aromatic essence" with alcohol and applied it to the upper lips of women with abnormal menstrual cycles and no current sexual relationship. The absorption or inhalation of this delightful concoction resulted in regular menstrual cycles in all ten women. The irregular menstrual cycles of six women in the control group, dabbed with only pure alcohol, remained irregular.

Another interesting phenomenon, long known to scientists and lay folks alike, is that women who work or live together tend to get their menstrual cycles at the same time. This is perhaps an indication that humans, like insects and some mammals, communicate subtly by sexual aromas known as pheromones.

*   *   *

Did you know that there was actually such an instrument as an orchidometer? Yes, and it measure orchids! Not the flowering type, but the type that most people refer to as the testicles.

*   *   *

Here's one that will make your palpebral fissure widen. The average weight of a Chinese man's testicles is 19.01 grams; however the average weight of a Dane's testicles is 42 grams—yes, I said 42 grams.

*   *   *

How about a Coke? A recent study released by Harvard Medical School may provide yet another method of contraception. Harvard researchers decided to test the effect of soft drinks on the viability of sperm.

In performing the study, they compared the effects that Diet Coke, Caffeine Free New Coke, New Coke, and Coke Classic had when poured into vials of viable sperm. Each individual type of Coke killed the little critters; however, there were significant differences in the effectiveness as well as the amount of time needed to annihilate the cohort.

New Coke proved to be the least effective of the five. Coke Classic was the go-getter of the group. It actually killed

New Coke proved to be the least effective of the five. Coke Classic was the go-getter of the group. It actually killed sperm five times faster than New Coke. Although the Coca-Cola Company refuses to endorse their product as a spermicidal agent, perhaps there is a new use as well as an explanation for the old Coca Cola douche.

* * *

An ounce of water weighs about 28 grams. A "junior" tampon is one that absorbs 6 grams or less of water in a standardized test; in contrast, "super-plus" absorbency tampons will absorb 12-15 grams. (Note: the higher the absorbency quotient the greater the risk for toxic shock syndrome. For each 1 gram increase in tampon absorbency, the risk increases 37%.)

The precursor to today's sanitary napkin can be attributed to French Army nurses during World War I. They discovered that the cellulose material used for covering and absorbing blood from wounds also worked well for absorbing menstrual blood. So, they discarded the cloth pads they had been using and began using the dressing for their menstrual flow. After World War I, the Kimberly Clark Corporation, who had supplied the U.S. Army with bandages, had an oversupply of bandage material and didn't know what to do with it. Someone in the corporation heard that the French Army nurses had put the bandages to good use. Kimberly Clark adopted the idea, and the "sanitary pad" became available for commercial use in 1921. Kimberly Clark chose the name "Kotex" as the designation for the firs disposable sanitary napkin, and it was followed shortly by "Modess" by Johnson and Johnson.

Tampons hit the market in 1933 amid much controversy, ridicule, scorn, and the misconception that inserting the tampon would "deflower" all of the virgins of the world.

* * *

A significant relationship exists between sexual behavior, hormone levels, and menstrual cycle length. This is most likely related to the sexual scent (pheromones) of the male. Women who have regular weekly heterosexual activity have menstrual cycles averaging 29 days in length. In contrast, women who are celibate or engage in sporadic (less than once a week) sexual activity, have lower levels of estradiol and a high frequency of irregular cycles. This link between consistent sexual activity (weekly) and high estradiol levels was also found in perimenopausal women. In fact, hot flashes and sexual activity are inversely related to one another. The more sexual activity, the fewer the hot flashes experienced. As a corollary, the more sexually active the perimenopausal woman remains, the milder the menopause.

The bottom line is—the more regular the sexual activity, the more regular the menstrual cycle. Regular menstrual cycles correlated with normal fertility patterns, whereas shorter cycles or longer cycles reflect a greater potential for fertility problems.

Does this hold true for men? Apparently there is definitely a "fertility" advantage in men as well. Men with weekly coital activity have higher sperm counts—not only is the quantity increased, but the quality is increased as well.

So, sexual activity on a weekly basis not only "primes the pump" so to speak, but makes it pregnant as well.

*   *   *

Another interesting fact observed in various studies related to fertility is that a delayed age at first coitus may be a contributing factor to infertility. It appears as if the first coital activity needs to be within seven years of the onset of menarche for optimal fertility.

*   *   *

MEDICAL MINUTIAE

intercourse. The rationale of course, was that the abdominal muscle contractions caused by sneezing could push sperm out of the vagina.

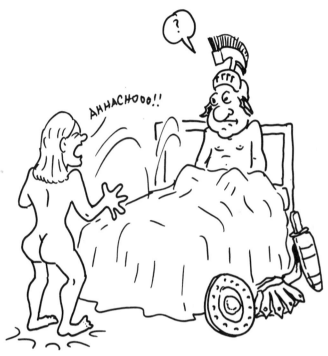

*   *   *

AUDIO CASSETTES BY BARB BANCROFT

If you have been to her seminars, you already know how she captivates participants. If you haven't, then you need to hear her tapes.

Audio Cassettes	APPROX. TIME	PRICE
Neuro for the Not-So-Neuro-Minded	4.5 Hours 4 Tapes	$40.00
Interpretation of Laboratory Tests	4.5 Hours 3 Tapes	$30.00
Endocrine Update*	4.5 Hours 3 Tapes	$30.00
Immunology Simplified	1 Hour 1 Tape	$10.00
Immunology — Update & Overview	5 Hours 4 Tapes	$40.00
Pediatric Physical Assessment	4.5-5 Hours 3 Tapes	$30.00
Journey Through the GI Tract	4.5-5 Hours 4 Tapes	$40.00
Osteoporosis	1 Hour 1 Tape	$10.00
WBC and Differential	1 Hour 1 Tape	$10.00
Shipping & Handling	1-2 Tapes $2.50	
Additional Tape(s) S&H	1-2 Tapes $1.00	
	TOTAL	

Please make check or money order payable to: CPP Associates, PO Box 14870, Chicago, Illinois 60614 (312) 477-8750.

Credit Cards accepted for orders over $25. Allow 2-4 weeks for delivery.
❑ Visa   ❑ MasterCard

Card No. _____ Exp. Date _____

Name _____

Address _____

City _____ ST _____ ZIP _____

PATHOPHYSIOLOGY PERSPECTIVES
...A MONTHLY NEWSLETTER FOR HEALTH CARE PROFESSIONALS

Pathophysiology Perspectives is a monthly newsletter written specifically to update health care professionals on current clinical topics. Each issue provides a comprehensive overview and update of one specific clinical entity. Examples:

- Update and Overview of Coronary Artery Disease in Women
- Inflammatory Bowel Disease
- Peptic Ulcer Disease
- Heparin-Induced Thrombocytopenia

In addition, each issue contains current updates on *Nutritional Nuggets, Treatment Updates, Journal Article Reviews,* and the ever popular, humorous antidotes in *Medical Minutiae.*

The cost of the 1995 annual individual subscription is $22.00; an institutional subscription (hospital, office, nursing school, agency) is $35.00. All subscriptions will begin with the January issue of the current year. Previous issues may also be purchased for $2.00 + postage and handling. (.75 for first issue and .25 for each additional issue). Please see reverse side for a list of 1994 issues.

*Please make check or money order payable to:
  CPP Associates
  PO Box 14870
  Chicago, Illinois 60614
  (312) 477-8750

Name _____

Address _____

City _____ *St* _____ *Zip* _____

Phone (_____ *)* _____

☐ Please send a sample copy. I have enclosed $2.00

☐ Please find my enclosed check or money order for $22.00 (Individual). $35.00 (institutional) one year subscription.

☐ Please send previous issues checked on the reverse side. I have enclosed $2.00 for each plus .75 for the 1st issue and .25 for each additional issue postage and handling.

1994 Pathophysiology Perspectives

January 1994: Peptic Ulcer Disease; Pharmacology Update; Nutritional Nuggets; Medical Minutiae

February 1994: Inflammatory Bowel Disease; Current Article Summaries; Treatment Updates; Medical Minutiae, Treatment One-Liners; Smoking and Surgery

March 1994: HIV Infection; What's Different in Women? Medical Minutiae; Neurology Update; Cardio-Vascular Update; Questions and Answers; Oncology Update; Diagnostic Trends; The Evaluation of Postoperative Fever

April/May 1994: Atrial Fibrillation; Cardiology Update; Neurology Update; Osteoporosis Update; Physical Diagnosis Tidbits; Diabetes Update; AIDS Update

June 1994: Inflammation and Immunity; Treatment One-Liners; Exercise and the Inner Ear; IV Steroids and Sickle Cell Disease; Passive Smoking; Aspirin Therapy; Tick-Borne Disease; Medical Minutiae

July 1994: STD Update — Herpes Genitalia; Geriatric Pearls; Nutritional Nuggets; AIDS Update; Treatement Update; Medical Minutiae; Neurology Updates

August 1994: Rheumatoid Arthritis — New Insights; Nutritional Nuggets; Medical Minutiae, Neurology Updates

September 1994: Hantavirus — Overview and Update; Treatment Update; Nutritional Nuggets; Medical Minutiae.

October/November 1994: Environmental Estrogens; Update on Women's Heal Issues; TV or not TV — That is the Question; Nutritional Nuggets; Medical Minutiae; Treatment Update; Physical Diagnosis Tidbits

December 1994: The Effects of Environmental Estrogens on Male Fertility; Torsemide — a New Loop Diuretic; Treatment One-Liners; Medical Minutiae; Nutritional Nuggets; Women's Health Issues.

Order Extra Copies for Friends and Co-Workers

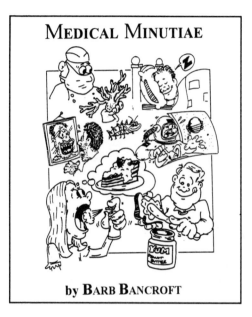

Please send me _____ copies of *Medical Minutiae*

Published by Willoworks Publishing. ISBN #0-945115-02-4. **$9.95**

Sales tax: Please add 8.75% for orders from Illinois
Shipping: $2.00 for the first book and 75¢ for each additional book. Allow four to six weeks for delivery.
Payments: Make check or money order payable to: Willoworks Publishing, PO Box 14870. Chicago, Illinois 60614

Credit Cards: Accepted for orders over $25.00.

☐ Visa ☐ MasterCard

Card No. _____ Exp. Date _____

Name _____

Address _____

City _____ ST _____ ZIP _____

Phone (_____) _____

Signature _____

(For credit card orders)

Also from Willoworks Publishing...For everyone who has a love/hate relationship with their car...

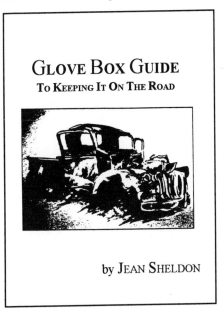

GLOVE BOX GUIDE
TO KEEPING IT ON THE ROAD

by JEAN SHELDON

An information filled guide for anyone who drives a car and has not totally adjusted to the world of "Self Serve Stations." Don't miss the mystery: *Who is Jack, and why is he in my trunk?*; *Unraveling the secret of jumper cables;* and the excitement of: *Handling a high speed blow-out.*Order your copy today!

Published by Willoworks Publishing. ISBN# 0-945115-01-6 **$8.95.**

Please send me _____ copies of *Glovebox Guide.*

Name: _____

Address: _____

City: _____ State: _____ Zip: _____

Credit Card # _____ Exp. Date _____

Signature _____ Phone _____

Sales tax: Please add 8.75% for order from Illinois
Shipping: $2.00 for the first book and 75¢ for each additional book. Allow four to six weeks for delivery.
Payments: Please make check or money order payable to: Willoworks Publishing, PO Box 14870. Chicago, Illinois 60614

EARTHSHINE

EARTHSHINE
DAVID YOUNG

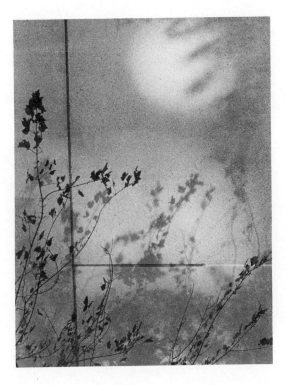

WESLEYAN UNIVERSITY PRESS
MIDDLETOWN, CONNECTICUT

"The Moon-Globe" and "Nine Deaths" appeared
originally in *Quarry West*.

Title page photograph by John Theilgard

All inquiries and permissions requests should be addressed
to the Publisher, Wesleyan University Press, 110 Mt. Vernon
Street, Middletown, Connecticut 06457.

Distributed by Harper & Row Publishers, Keystone Industrial
Park, Scranton, Pennsylvania 18512.

LIBRARY OF CONGRESS
CATALOGING-IN-PUBLICATION DATA
Young, David, 1936-
Earthshine / David Young.
ISBN 0-8195-2147-7   ISBN 0-8195-1148-x (pbk.)
I. Title.
PS3575.078E2   1988   87-21183
811'.54—dc19   CIP

Manufactured in the United States of America

FIRST EDITION

WESLEYAN POETRY

for Georgia
and
for Chloe

CONTENTS

ONE

The Moon-Globe

This small tin model of the moon,
gift of a friend, tipped on its stand,
is one of the featured and featureless
things that survive you now.

It's mapped, but not in relief:
one can see and study, but not feel,
the craters and mountain ranges.
Sometimes I rub the missing wrinkles.

There's no dark side to this moon.
No light one either.
Just enough gloss to reflect
a smudge of daylight on its gray-blue surface.

I move it from desk to bedside,
giving my grief a little spin,
putting the surface, which ought to be rough,
against my shaved and moony cheek.

TWO

Nine Deaths

"Cancer is a series of deaths."
Georgia Newman

1. *Surgery*

Late April. You've just learned
they will cut away your breast, or part of it.

We've cried,
discussed statistics,
told our children and friends. For relief
and a little privacy
we drive out
to West Road
south of the reservoir,
and walk in the green spring evening
hearing cows and birds, watching leafing trees.

"The world's so beautiful," I say. Or is that you?
We hold hands.
This is a death, the first,
and we can bear it.

Not too bad.
Not good, though.

2. *Liver Scan*

It's summer now. Your radiation's over
and you're to start
chemotherapy:
"poisoning the body
to poison the disease," in one view,
but a way to buy some time and hope for most.
In the last conference at the Cleveland Clinic
before we leave for six weeks in Vermont
we get bad news:

7

a liver scan
shows two spots,
metastases,
the cancer erupting in a new place.

The chemo will have to be
much more severe: you'll have nausea, fatigue,
you'll lose your lovely hair.
I hold your hand
tightly
as the doctor talks.
We both feared this.
The statistics he gives
are still encouraging
but hope has shrunk.
This is another death. We live
inside a tighter circle now.

All day we drive east.
Since Margaret, with us,
doesn't know and you don't want to worry her,
nothing is said.
Whenever I glance at you
your face is peaceful.
We listen to music, read the scenery,
fold and unfold our maps.
Oh this is a death, all right
as we head up
toward the Green Mountains
clinging to two hopes:
recovery, hardly likely,
and a good long stand-off in your body
between the cancer and the chemicals
that will start to weaken your heart.

You have
a little more
than nineteen months
to live.

3. Indefinitely

Now there's an interlude of nearly a year
in which there's no death, just some dying,
and most of it bearable.
Vermont is peaceful, Breadloaf is lively
in just the right way. We go to Burlington
for treatments, shop for a wig,
bring back fresh bagels.
Walks, reading, visits from friends,
at our small cabin in the woods.
You audit a course on *Ulysses*,
work on an article, your last one.
We don't have sex as often:
you feel fragile and the chemo
makes your vagina dry,
but we feel close and, often, happy,
lucky to have each other for the time,
and our two children, half adults,
one with us, raising a robin in a box,
the other at home with a job,
playing at man of the house.

By the end of the summer you're bald
and we're off for four months in England,
me to teach, you to research and write
and visit museums as you can.

You're not as able as you hoped.
Everywhere in the city

you need to take my arm,
shaky in traffic and crowds,
tiring easily.

You stay home a lot and read.
You hate the wig and tend to wear
scarves and bandannas,
whose look, peasant or gypsy, I grow to love.
We get to a lot of theater,
exhibits, side trips to Bath, Stratford,
the Lake District.
Sometimes your appetite is good,
sometimes you can't take much
except some tea and oatmeal.
Sometimes you throw up, again and again.

We know it's the price we pay
for holding off the disease
and you don't complain.

You don't complain about London either
but I can tell
how glad you are
to get back home.

Now they change the regimen.
After a year, people on this one
start to have massive heart failure.

You ask your Cleveland doctor
how long you'll be on this new set of drugs.
As long as they work, he tells you,
to keep those liver spots from spreading.
And then? And then a new set.

And how long on chemotherapy?
Indefinitely, he says.

It comes across us both,
a sickening dawn that we saw coming:
we can't expect to beat the disease.
It's June. Ripe summer has set in again.
This is a death.

4. Seizure

One August night, after a bad movie
(*Indiana Jones and the Temple of Doom*),
you wake me with your movements.
Thinking you need to go to the bathroom,
I try to help you up, but you fall, helpless,
hitting your face on the night-table.
Then come convulsions. Then unconsciousness.
Is this a stroke? Some new disease?
Shaking, I summon the ambulance
and they take you to Emergency.
You have another seizure there. They drug you,
    admit you,
and send me home at 3 a.m. Next day,
a CAT scan confirms the doctor's hunch:
two little tumors in the brain.
These can be treated by radiation, we're assured.
The real risk continues in the liver.
You can have radiation to the skull and still
help me drive Margaret to college.
Gradually, gingerly,
we move back into our routines.
You have no memory of your seizure.
You often ask me about it.
I remember everything,

too vividly: the horror of your fall,
my helplessness, your absence in convulsions
and unconsciousness.
It's taken me three months
to tell this part of the story.
That's how I know what a death it is.
Almost the biggest one.
And yet our lives go on.
You have a new doctor, whom you like the best
of all of them. You're back at work.
Like Indiana Jones you seem to have had
one more miraculous escape.
Down in my heart, I know different.

5. Lung Spots

September. A chest x-ray
that looked all right at first
is taken again and studied further.
There are two spots on the lung.

This isn't so serious, we're told.
If the spots don't grow, the new chemo's working,
and it will be easier to monitor.
The liver is still
the biggest danger.

Neither one of us, for a while,
can admit to what we're thinking:
now the disease has turned up
four separate places. How long
till it spreads to yet another?
And when it turns up in the blood, the bone,
the other breast . . .

I know how much this sets you back
by how long it takes you to tell
your father and your children.

I don't know how much
you cry in the bathroom
or when I'm not around.

This is a little death, but it goes deep.

6. Anemia

You keep on going to work.
Morning after morning,
dropping you off,
watching your slow movements,
I feel my heart
crack into contrary parts:
admiration for your courage,
sorrow for your slow decline.

Christmas comes, a loved one,
but you are weak and can't eat much.
You sleep a lot and we both pretend
your lack of appetite is temporary,
a matter of adjusting to the chemo
and learning what is palatable.

Oh eating is death and hunger is death,
and I don't know, or won't admit it.
We drift through January, a rugged month,
and I make soups, brown rice and junkets.
Somehow the things you ate as a child,

your mother's bridge club casseroles
and thirties cooking,
help you most. You dwindle,
and we both try not to notice.
Finally, one early February night,
your breathing grows terribly labored
and next day
I take you to the doctor.

You're anemic, she tells us,
and some blood transfusions will help.
She admits you to the hospital.
I'm relieved
to have you in competent hands.
But there's something ominous in this.
You sense it more than I do.
Midafternoon, the last time we talk,
you cry a little. I try to cheer you up
and promise to make the calls
to friends and family
to say you're in the hospital
and hoping to get out
healthy and pink again
in a day or two.

7. *Heart Failure*

Your heart fails during the transfusion.
Weakened by medication, it can't drive
your damaged lungs.
Your breathing stops.
They rush you to Intensive Care
and manage to revive you,
hooking you up to a breathing machine
that helps you—makes you?—go on living.

You never regain consciousness.
Three days we watch beside your bed,
talking to you, whispering, pleading.
I summon the family,
chat with the minister,
go through the motions of normal life,
try to endure
the pity of watching you kept alive
by a mindless apparatus.

I want to let you go. I want to keep you.

Where has your beauty gone,
your gaze, your poise and animation?
What or who am I standing beside?
What ears hear my whispers of love?

8. Unplug the Respirator
This is the doctor's idea.
A scan shows you've probably been gone,
brain-dead,
since the heart first stopped.

Is this then the moment of death?
This is the eighth of nine.

9. She's Like a Painting / Bless Her Heart
At the last you look composed,
unhooked, released, at peace,
as we come in groups of two and three
to take our leave of you.

I can touch and kiss you again,
though your waxy stillness
tells me I'm kissing your husk.

My mind shoots like a bobsled
back through the whole course of the illness.
Once again, arm in arm,
summoning courage,
we are walking out of the Cleveland Clinic . . .

One last look for us.
"She's like a painting," whispers Margaret.
And that is true.

"Bless her heart," says my simple mother,
twice,
and those words are oddly right.
That damaged heart
that kept you going
and gave you strength to face your death . . .

You're like a painting.

Bless your heart.

10. Coda

Your deaths are over.
My dreams begin.

In the first you are wearing a striped blouse
and vomiting in the kitchen sink.
I watch your back from a helpless distance.

In the second, helping you move to a chair
at some social gathering,
I realize you are lifeless
like a mummy or a dummy.

In the third, I arrive running, late,
for some graveside service.
You are waiting in the crowd, impatient and withdrawn.
But then you embrace me.
What a relief to touch you again!

These dreams are not your visits,
just my clumsy inventions.
I live in an empty house
with wilting flowers and spreading memories
and my own heart
that hollows and fills.
I'm addressing you
and you can't hear me.
If you can, you don't need
to be told this story.
I need to tell it to myself
until I can stand to hear it.

And you're not here
except in the vaguest ways.

Were you the hawk
that followed us back
from your memorial service
that brilliant winter day?

Are you the rabbit
I keep seeing
that's tamer than it should be?

I wish I could believe it.
You're none of these things or all of them.

What does Montale say?
Words from the oven, words from the freezer,
that's what poetry is.

This is neither.
This is an empty house and a heart
that hollows and fills, hollows and fills

Chloe Hamilton Young, 1927–1985

THREE

Poem in Three Parts

To Halley's Comet

Thumbsmear, figment, dust-and-ice-ball portent,
what the Chinese called "broomstar" and the Greeks
named for its gassy hair, a halo of plasma
kinked and knotted by magnetic fields: comet
my father will see twice, I'll offer this to you,
since it deals with gravity, motion and light
and you can mean all three,
                    though you don't know
Earth's lovely pull, only the sun's fierce yoyo game,
and you can't move, except along your long, looped track,
and you can't see the hues and gleams
our light-show throws around, just our own blue glow
in the proton wind—still, I'd like to mark your passage
by this small celebration, twined with my own life,
of where we live and why we tend to love it.

I. Broken Field Running

1.

What stands on one leg at night?
staggers and stalks?

Oedipus never heard the whole riddle—
the Sphinx held something back . . .

What feels its legs turn to one root
twisting down into humus and duff?

—Even today, in modern Thebes,
 somebody building a house
 will find in the excavation
 so many statues and funeral pots
 the project turns into a dig—

Oh cities and cities of the dead . . .

What made the Laius family limp?

                    It's hard
to free your foot from that dreamy earth-pull
and you drag it, leaving a seed-grave.

2.

Eighteen-sixty-four:
Hopkins sketches a drowned rat
floating past on the Isis.

Hears voices from a well,
piping and whistling.

Decides he had better be a priest.

—If I sign up with the sky-god
can I still do broken field running?

3.

When Hare first heard about Death
he gnashed his teeth, went to his lodge,
and started screaming.

My aunts and uncles mustn't die!

His thoughts went up to the cliffs and they started to crumble,
crawled across rocks and they shattered,
went down in the earth where everything stilled and stiffened,
glanced at the sky and birds crashed down, dead thoughts.

He went to his lodge, lay down
and wrapped himself in his blanket.

Earth isn't big enough.
It will be hard, all those dead,
and not enough earth to hold them!

And he lay there, wrapped in his blanket.

4.

And isn't the earth our goddess?
When we run through a muddy field
don't we step in her clutching hands?

Weren't the male sky-gods
our dream of escape from her? Isn't
gravity
mother-love,
apron-string, homing instinct?

To deny autochthony!
                    Going up in smoke,
the rising-trick of the kite,
                    the swaddled astronaut
knifing his lifeline and tumbling away
                    into a motherless dark . . .

In a basket
hung from my cruising balloon
I find
my gaze
pulled to her fields
all fenced and winter-fallow.

Today she is sound asleep, it's bitter February,
even the birds have abandoned
this white and star-crossed air,
and I can talk about her some.

I know I touched her at Castlerigg
in cloud-wet Cumberland—
not the stone circle so much
as the barely visible furrows
left by the Dark-Age plows,
marks of her longevity.

Cremate us! we plead, dreaming escape again, but the smoke
melts into the water cycle, her old prayer wheel, and the ashes,
even dumped at sea,
drift in the currents of her cold and giant love.

5.

Nineteen-oh-five.
Joyce in Trieste
is writing "The Dead."
Nora and Giorgio are asleep.
Something about Rome,
maybe all those catacombs
or the sleepy look of ruins,
reminded him of Ireland
and its loose hordes of ghosts.

He writes the final sentences
and his Gabriel gives in
to the vast chthonic pull
while Joyce imagines he
himself goes free. Not so.
All Trieste's asleep—
the snow is general
all over Europe.
Joyce had a mother too.

6.

A last tune
on this bone flute
as the breath goes up and out
and most of the rest of what we were,
grateful and biodegradable,
sinks in her huge embrace
muttering some of her names,
gravity-heavy, muddy and dazed,
spread-eagled on the battlefield
curled in the passage grave
cool in the miles of catacomb
shake hands, shake hands, shake hands . . .

7.

Bat-shadows
hoof prints
"pool and rut-peel patches"

all her marks and mottles

the garden, the lawn, the tennis court, lawn again,
woods!
       trees fallen, tilted, upright.
   tangles of vine and brush
   spawn pools, fungus erupting from trunks
wood you can crumble, leaf-pulp

a muskrat
      skips into the creek, dives out of sight
       a turtle dozes coldly on a snag

this is her realm
moss
slabs of trickling stone and tiny ferns
deep caves
shadow people slipping out of sight.

At the caves at Font-de-Gaume
where the deer and bison float
on bulges in the rockface
I felt the way
I feel in a cathedral.

No, better:
closer to home.

8.

My garret in New Haven,
down by the newspaper plant—
when trains went by below
everything would tremble.

The first time it happened
I thought I had the shakes
but then I saw that the pictures,
the light bulb, the cheap clock,
and the tarnished mirror over the dresser
were trembling too.

Spring evenings I sat by the window
melancholy as a bear
and once I was so ecstatic
I had a vision: an albatross
settling on my chest.

But mostly it was incessant study
and knowing too little about the earth
and the periodic rumbling from the trains
and nothing for the mirror to reflect on.

9.

Nearly the middle of March, snow everywhere
and I'm watching three winter finches,
"sparrows dipped in raspberry juice,"
take turns at the neighbor's feeder.

Winter won't let go.
Under our pine a half-starved possum
chews sunflower seeds,
watched by disgusted squirrels.

My body sees all this
but my spirit is somewhere else
crossing potato fields in Poland
merged with some poor fugitive
pursued by the S.S.
forty-two years ago.

Later, I know, they will torture us.

Crouched in a hazel copse,
freckled with light and panting.

What causes we have to be speechless—
this century, shuddering toward its close,
has worked and twisted us
until there seems to be nothing
but muteness or scream . . .

10.

I shake my liar's head.

I've never been in Poland.

What is the etymology of torment?

Why has the possum been willing
to come so close to the house?

I know I imagined that albatross . . .

What will the S.S. men
do with my mud-caked shoes?

"Listen," I try to tell them,
"fill these with good black dirt
and plant a seed in each."

Plow us all in and try again.

Rolling toward spring, this earth,
this March of nineteen-eighty-four.

January–March 1984

II. Dancing in the Dark

1.

In an old scrub-orchard
a mile or two from Everyville
I see a naked couple
maybe it's you and me
around the end of August
doing something by moonlight
that could involve a search
for love or buried treasure
or something good to eat
it's just too dim from here
to tell exactly what
but I know our movements make
a lot of sense to us . . .

A line and a turn and a new line
and something fresh each time
and the lie spins round on its toe
and is, by God, the truth.

2.

The reservoir once more, on a still evening,
great gold and purple doings in the west.
Things are so still just now that it takes minutes
to pick out any motion: a ripple spreading slowly
from where a bluegill rose, a faint stir in the milkweeds,
nothing much livelier than a rusting Plymouth . . .

Motion's a lie? Rest is a bigger one.
I can take movement and all that it implies,
the skid and stub of fact, fits, fists and shakes,
heartmurmurs, toe and heel, love and its bristling opposites,
muskrat ramble and turkey strut, these gnats
making formations so complicated
they might not be patterns at all. I think
I'll move my bones around this shore
while there's still light to see.

3.

October three. Jade-green, Plum Creek slides by,
pocked with small rings and bubbles
                twin-rimmed circles
that spread and overlap and coast the current.

            And the face in the tree is howling.

        I pace across the grass. Curled copper leaves
are half-entreating hands with cupped
                reflections of the day.
The dice jump in the box. Rain falls.

            And the face in the tree is howling.

        Glass beads line the undersides of twigs. A sparrow
dives in a juniper bush, then fires
                out the other side, intent upon
a pattern of his own in this good rain—

            And the face in the tree is howling.

4.

"Rabbits in Alabama hop," I wrote in 1963,
happy enough between two deaths: a summer friend
and a November president. New-married, love-sheathed,
I could feel the planet's wobble and bounce
as I walked my dog through weeds and stubble
grasshoppers spraying in every direction
so that I called myself "hub of a wheel,"
teasing my sturdy little ego
tingling along like a streetcar,
not yet in the undertow of fatherhood,
soft shoe in the cornfield, dust mote dance,
loving the action I saw spread out—
a map of this generous, jumping-bean country.

5.

Industrial sky this afternoon, gray rags
swabbing a dim chrome button.
I seem to hear a drum and tambourine.

The branches are wiggling in thundery wind
and the last few leaves, washed from the trees,
sail through my line of sight.

Everything's moving. We never know that.
Molecules vibrate in the solid rock
out of our ken, an act of faith.

Even if helium freezes, Margaret tells me,
it's two degrees above absolute zero
and there's movement, however sluggish.

In the Milky Way's heart a magnet pulses.
Holy Ghost, spraying neutrinos and gamma rays,
come closer to our stethoscope!

+

Edmund Spenser has a headache
from trying to write *The Faerie Queene*:
Has come to court a little tipsy.

Watching the regal bitch
whirl through a wild lavolta
her face a grinning, red-wigged skull,

"I hear the music of the spheres,"
he mutters to himself,
"and it's the dance of death."

But life and death are tango partners, Ned,
mincing through figures, cheek to cheek,
we cannot hope to read.

                    More leaves spin by,
minnows off the willows, oak-brown batwings.
And the trees rock in the giant pulse. And hold.

6.

In Finney Chapel Ivo Pogorelich
is playing Beethoven's C-Minor Sonata.
Now it's November. Gusts of rain
hammer the walls and roof. For a second
the pianist's fingers match the cascade
and he smiles, a very faint smirk.

Lightning splits off grins outside.
Dark leers. Trees crack.

But here the piano dances gingerly.
Rain-dance. Didn't this smile cross
the composer's face as he scanned the score,
hummed a bar, sipped his coffee,
and sneezed in the sunlight? Sure.
Listening to the downpour? Sure.

7.

A London Saturday. One year ago.
C. and I walk through the V and A,
happy to study replicas. Half a mile off
the Irish Republican Army
has car-bombed a street next to Harrods.
Blood
and broken glass
and a strange hush. Elsewhere,
a waiter drizzles oil on a salad.
In our flat near Baker Street
my wife reads, turning pages.
Bright fibers rim a shawl. Pink candles
infuse a churchy gloom.
Smell of ammonia from somewhere.
A guard yawns. A madman squints.
Hung by its feet,
a pheasant sways in a butcher's window.
Leaves blow in the park.
Time bleeds.
Holly bushes glitter.

Once again I do not know
how this can be turned into words
and held steady
even for a moment:
it slides across your eye
and flickers in your mind.

You look up from the page.

8.

Listening to the Verdi Requiem
while the dog whimpers in her sleep
both of us in a patch of winter sunlight
and I feel my tear-ducts prickle once again—
oh all this being mortal, keeping brave,
and trying to stay on course for X,
like the blue jay arriving at his cry
or the prima ballerina
sailing into the audience
here and gone, flesh and word,
the boxcar turning slowly in the water
and settling on the bottom of the lake.

9.

I'm watching the brown tangle of tomato vines
in our December garden. They don't move.

If everything is dancing
even beyond our senses
and even if it's mad and random,
that must help explain consciousness,
perched in the body, bird in a tree,
chirps, preens, looks wildly about,
even when dozing is alert,
metabolism racing,
beady-eye, singsong, flutter and shit—

If consciousness could match the body better
and be a bear
and even hibernate?

Oh then it would miss fine things!

On Christmas Eve it snowed
as if we lived in a greeting card.
The snow blowing off the roof
and through the backyard floodlight
as we watched from around the fire
made intricate patterns: scallops, loops,
tangles and alphabets. We're seeing the wind,
we realized, dressed
in powdery snow. Nothing to worship,
but something to wonder at,
a little epiphany, in season.

Pigeons in Buffalo, Holub told me,
can hear the Concorde landing in New York.
So what do we think we know? All of our dancing
is done in the dark, on the ceiling, the page, over the gorge
on the bridge of rotten rope and sturdy instinct.

I think I did worship that wind.

Belief is a move from branch to branch.
It doesn't much matter where you perch.
You may be hearing the Concorde. You may not.

10.

And yesterday a red-tailed hawk
killed and ate a mourning dove
in the middle of a snowstorm
in our back yard. For five minutes
that made a violent, bobbing center
for everything else in sight:
the swirl of flakes, the pine boughs
    humped with snow,
the smaller birds who fled,
our curious eyes and breath.
And then the center shifted.

Any still point we choose
is relative to observation;
the planet rolled ahead, dragging
its dead and gorgeous moon,
great storms shot up on the sun,
whole galaxies stood by and gleamed
and maybe an owl in a hollow tree
two hundred yards away from us
swiveled his head and blinked
hearing the little death.
The hawk rose up, his tail a flare of rust,
and a sprinkle of torn feathers
began to blow across the snow
till we could see no more.

September 1984–February 1985

44

III. The Light Show

1.

Light breaks, the Welshman said
where no sun shines. And Uncle Ezra spoke
of light that was not of the sun.
On Metaphor Hill I met my match.

A butterfly hovers at the windowpane.
She's gone. That was my sunshine.
Or thereabouts. I find no light
except what was, an afterglow of love,

and then this stuff that wags and pants
across the day. Good light. Good dog.
Ten lines to sunset. Later on
by starlight I may meet her?

Don't I wish. "His wife's dead,"
they say. "He must be stunned." Indeed.
Light breaks. I break. Good egg.
Good Doctor Astrov meets his match.

2.

Today the April light is fizzing.
The wind is blowing chunks of it around:
it oils pine needles, runs up tree trunks
and spreads in clumps across the grass.
The grackles struggle darkly to resist it,
but it glosses their necks with purple and green
and slicks their beaks. I too
feel misery start to slip away—against my grain
I'm hoisted into this giant light-machine
and swept away. My silver pen
skates on the yellow paper, my fingernails glow
my eyes glisten with tears and pleasure.
A huge willow has fallen in my yard,
victim of wind. But today the other trees
are holding themselves up like song into a sky
that's blue with a radiance no one could imagine.

Gaze of Apollo that kindled Rilke
even in a headless torso.
                              Maybe *because*
it was piecemeal.
                    We need shadows,
smoked glass, spiritual parasols. Caravaggio
knew how contingent light is, how
it comes from the wrong side, lighting
lovers and murderers indifferently.
                                    Well, we *are*
star-ash. Residue. Cooling sizzle
from an old mayhem of the sun.

Galactic epigones and afterlights.

And we love light *and* shade,
color and just a little dazzle.
If I called you a feather on the breath of God,
you'd want to know what color? Right!
Different if it were white, in thin noon breeze,
or black, zigzagging through dusk's pines,
or brown, at dawn, upon an olive river . . .

Rodin, I learn,
liked his wax version of *The Gates of Hell*
for its "blond shadows." Who doesn't love
light's pleasing accidents and glances?
The casual star my dropped keys make,
the wren's flight, a molecule of deity
cut loose, both particle and wave
chaos across the retina, then night,
scaring the daylights out of the west.

And Proust remembered a restaurant front
"glazed and streaming with light."
I think of your lit skin, your limbs and breasts
when we made love by firelight. It may be
that all my poems celebrating light
have had your beauty as their subtext.
But I'll not hand the grief-cup round . . .

Edward Lear, the epileptic,
disappointed painter, found
the English daylight fickle:
"a tree is black one minute,
the next it's yellow, and the 3rd green;
so that were I to finish any part
the whole would be all spots—
a sort of Leopard Landscape."
He wrestled his easel back to the studio.

Light the Leopard. Springs in the new year.
Us he devours? But the wren lives on.
Lear is remembered for his limericks,
his ready nonsense. Spotted and inconstant,
we love the life we say we yearn to lose.

5.

Light in the mountains—the Andes, in this case—
is hard to know. It visits gorges
absent-mindedly, lingers on reddened peaks
leaves foregrounds shadowed black and backgrounds
bathed in brilliance. Light makes huge turns,
filling whole slopes and missing their neighbors,
a cataract switched on and off.

Here at Macchu Picchu
the daylight pulls away and up
leaving us in a darkened saucer.
All night two dogs
bark on and off at the knuckle-sized stars
and the sun comes back by brightening
beyond the rim of peaks.

Glaze of daylight. Clouds you can stroke,
sun that strokes you. A total eclipse
would be unbearable. Down in the gorge,
a steady roar from the little pewter river.
And then this neolithic city
strung like a harp, terracing the air,
carving the mountain light with mountain stone . . .

Neruda was here. Pretending
he was an Indian, hankering
to speak for a whole continent!
He might be looking down now
from that sun, rolling up his sleeves.
I raise my arm and shield my eyes.
Affectionate salute.

6.

Light in the ocean—I'm snorkeling
at the Equator, Hood Island, Galápagos,
in the sunken rim of a volcano—
is Vermeer-light, its workclothes

green undulating vestments, shot with salt.
It comes by streaks and ramps, in rings and stations,
angelfish seeming to burn from within,
snow-fall, tide-pull, quiet pandemonium.

I kick through coral shadows, lava tubes.
Sight picks out fish with yellow lips,
black dinner plates with glowing violet rims,
whole schools of tiny city lights, striped neckties . . .

A wave breaks: silver eggs cascade.
A seal twists by. Huge forces rinse me.
I ponder gardens, malachite and orange, while sorrow
slips from me and is vanquished in the currents.

7.

At our Midsummer party
we tried to have all kinds of light:
a bonfire, candles, Tahiti torches,
fireflies adding their dots on the dark;
we set off pinwheels, Roman candles,
brandished sparklers—and later, above embers,
we were content with starlight.
I was a little miserable. I thought
myself on the other shore of love;
the pinwheels were for the sun's renewal,
not for mine. My mind went back
to the sun's other birthday,
that Christmas Eve we read "The Dead"
and watched the snow in the floodlight.

Love makes the world precious? Yes,
and loss of ego brings on love,
snow sifting off the roof
to blow where the night wind takes it . . .

8.

Georgia,
even your snapshot
fills me with singing light.
You're holding Tom, you're standing next to
an amiable priest who came to bless the fields.
You're looking out at the world with love and trust,
giving yourself, steady as a lamp.
The tears that filled me up
fill with light now:
mountain light, sea light,
midsummer light and Christmas light.
Refraction. Rilke spoke his hope:
"That this homely weeping might bloom."
And Tu Fu imagined the moonlight
drying the tear-tracks on two faces.
Whatever happens to me in this life,
including the blow that finally knocks me dead,
your light will remind me to love and praise,
the day coming up again,
the world enacting its own beginnings,
and everything moving in this earthshine.

9.

Earthrise: from its rubbled moon
I'm watching the sun's third planet.

It's blue and white, with flecks of brown and green.
Vast weather systems swirl and mottle it.
Moist, breathing through its fantastic
membrane of atmosphere,
it crowds my heart with love.

The world's suspended, Chekhov says,
on the tooth of a dragon. Even that tooth gleams.

I've come here to figure out how light
streams to the wheeling planet,
a solar blast, photons and protons,
and helps it live. Morowitz
and Lewis Thomas tell us
that energy from the sun
doesn't just flow to earth
and radiate away: "It is
thermodynamically inevitable
that it must rearrange
matter into symmetry,
away from probability,
against entropy,
lifting it, so to speak,
into a constantly changing
condition of rearrangement
and molecular ornamentation."

Which is how I got here, I suppose,
some rearranged matter
imagining and praising
"a chancy kind of order,"
always about to be chaos again,
"held taut
against probability
by the unremitting
surge of energy"
streaming out of the sun.

Behind, above, below me, stars:
countless suns with the same meaning!

Before me, leisurely as a peacock,
the turning earth.

10.

It's a late October afternoon:
warm winds and distant thunder.
Leaves catch the sunlight as they shower down.

Just over my outstretched fingertips
floats Emily Dickinson, horizontal spirit:
"See all the light, but see it slant,"
is what she seems to murmur.

I don't know. All through these months
I've been a well with two buckets:
one for grief and one for love.
Sometimes the daylight has bewildered me.

A day as bright and intricate as a crystal,
an afternoon that will not go away—
one of Time's strange suspensions.

The Gospel Lighthouse Church's lemon-yellow bus
says "Heaven Bound" up front. They feel they know.
Last night, what made me think
we are continuous with a noumenal world
was a sheet of blank paper in my midnight bedroom
rising and falling in a midnight breeze.

This afternoon my house
is flooded with late sunlight
and the next sheet of paper after this one
is white, and is for you.

March–October 1986

FOUR

The Portable Earth-Lamp

The planet on the desk, illuminated globe
we ordered for Bo's birthday,
sits in its lucite crescent, a medicine ball
of Rand McNally plastic. A brown cord
runs from the South Pole toward a socket.

It's mostly a night-light for the boys,
and it blanches their dreaming faces,
a blue sphere patched with continents,
mottled by deeps and patterned currents,
its capital cities bright white dots.

Our models: they're touching and absurd,
magical for both their truth and falsehood.

I like its shine at night. Moth-light.
I sleepwalk toward it, musing.
This globe's a bible, a bubble of myth-
light, a blue eye, a double
bowl: empty of all but its bulb and clever skin,
full of whatever we choose to lodge there.

I haven't been able to shake off all my grief,
my globe's cold poles and arid wastes,
the weight of death, disease and history.
But see how the oceans heave and shine,
see how the clouds and mountains glisten!

We float through space. Days pass.
Sometimes we know we are part of a crystal
where light is sorted and stored,
sharing an iridescence
cobbled and million-featured.

Oh tiny beacon in the hurting dark.
Oh soft blue glow.

OTHER BOOKS BY DAVID YOUNG

POEMS
Sweating Out the Winter
Boxcars
Work Lights: Thirty-two Prose Poems
The Names of a Hare in English
Foraging

TRANSLATIONS
Rilke, *Duino Elegies*
Four T'ang Poets
Valuable Nail: Selected Poems of Gunter Eich
(with Stuart Friebert and David Walker)
Miroslav Holub, *Interferon, or On Theater*
(with Dana Hábová)
Rilke, *Sonnets to Orpheus*
Neruda, *The Heights of Macchu Picchu*

CRITICISM
Something of Great Constancy:
The Art of
"A Midsummer Night's Dream"
The Heart's Forest: Shakespeare's Pastoral Plays
Troubled Mirror: A Study of Yeats's "The Tower"

ANTHOLOGIES
Twentieth Century Interpretations of "2 Henry IV"
A FIELD Guide to Contemporary Poetry and Poetics
(with Stuart Friebert)
The Longman Anthology of Contemporary American Poetry
(with Stuart Friebert)
Magical Realist Fiction (with Keith Hollaman)

About the Author

David Young is the author of five other books of poetry: *Sweating Out the Winter, Boxcars, Work Lights: Thirty-two Prose Poems, The Names of a Hare in English,* and *Foraging* (Wesleyan, 1986). He is also a translator of five books including *Sonnets to Orpheus* (Wesleyan, 1987). A professor of English at Oberlin College, Young received a B.A. from Carleton College (1958) and a Ph.D. from Yale in 1965. He edits *Field,* a literary magazine, and serves as an arbiter of *Field*'s translation series. He lives in Oberlin, Ohio.

About the Book

This book was composed on the Mergenthaler 202 in Baskerville, a contemporary rendering of a fine transitional typeface named for the eighteenth-century English printer John Baskerville. It was adapted for the 202 from the Linotype version by the Mergenthaler Corporation. The book was composed by G&S Typesetters of Austin, Texas, and designed and produced by Kachergis Book Design, Pittsboro, North Carolina.

ACQ-46665

2/14
gy

PS
3575
O78
E2
1988